HEALING
YOGA

'TO GROW TRULY AND BECOME REALLY HUMAN WE MUST
GO THROUGH THE LIFE PROCESS. SOME SUFFER MENTALLY,
EMOTIONALLY OR SPIRITUALLY; SOME GET HYPERTENSION AND
OTHERS GET ULCERS. THIS IS ALL PART OF OUR SCHOOLING
HERE ON EARTH. PARADOXICALLY, SOME OF US MUST GET SICK
TO LEARN ABOUT OURSELVES MORE FULLY AND COMPLETELY.'

Swami Satyananda Saraswati

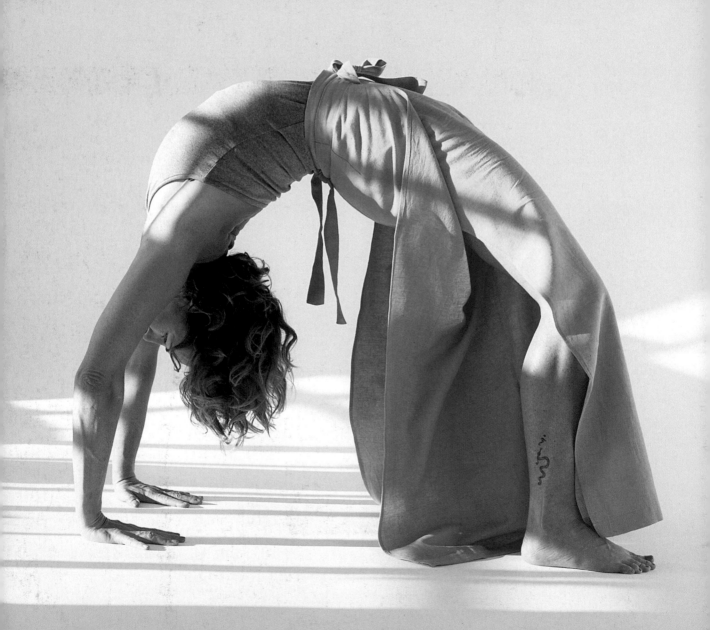

HEALING
YOGA

LIZ LARK and TIM GOULLET

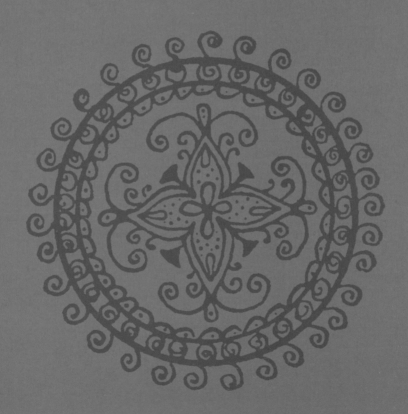

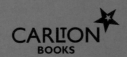

CARLTON
BOOKS

THIS IS A CARLTON BOOK

Text copyright © 2005 Liz Lark and Tim Goullet
Design and special photography copyright © 2005
Carlton Books Limited

This edition published by
Carlton Books Limited 2005
20 Mortimer Street
London W1T 3JW

ISBN 1 84442 778 1 (hardback)
ISBN 1 84442 511 8 (paperback)

Printed and bound in Dubai

Executive Editor: **Lisa Dyer**
Senior Art Editor: **Zoë Dissell**
Photographer: **Clare Park**
Designer: **Penny Stock**
Make-up Artist: **Sophia Atcha**
Copy Editor: **Kelly Thompson**
Production Controller: **Lisa French**
Models: **Sujata Banerjee, Lee Brindell, Tim Goullet,
Liz Lark, Tara Lee**

It is important to consult your doctor before commencing
any exercise programme. This is particularly the case if
you have a medical condition (including but not limited to
abnormal blood pressure or a back injury), have had surgery
recently or are pregnant and, even then, you should only
undertake these programmes with a well-trained teacher.
All instructions and warnings given in this book should be
read carefully. This book is not intended to replace personal
instruction or professional medical advice. The warnings listed
for some of the poses are guidelines only.

The author and publisher have made every effort to ensure
that all information is correct and up to date at the time of
publication. Neither the author or publisher can accept
responsibility for, or shall be liable for, any accident, injury, loss
or damage (including any consequential loss) that results from
using the ideas, information, procedures or advice offered in
this book.

contents

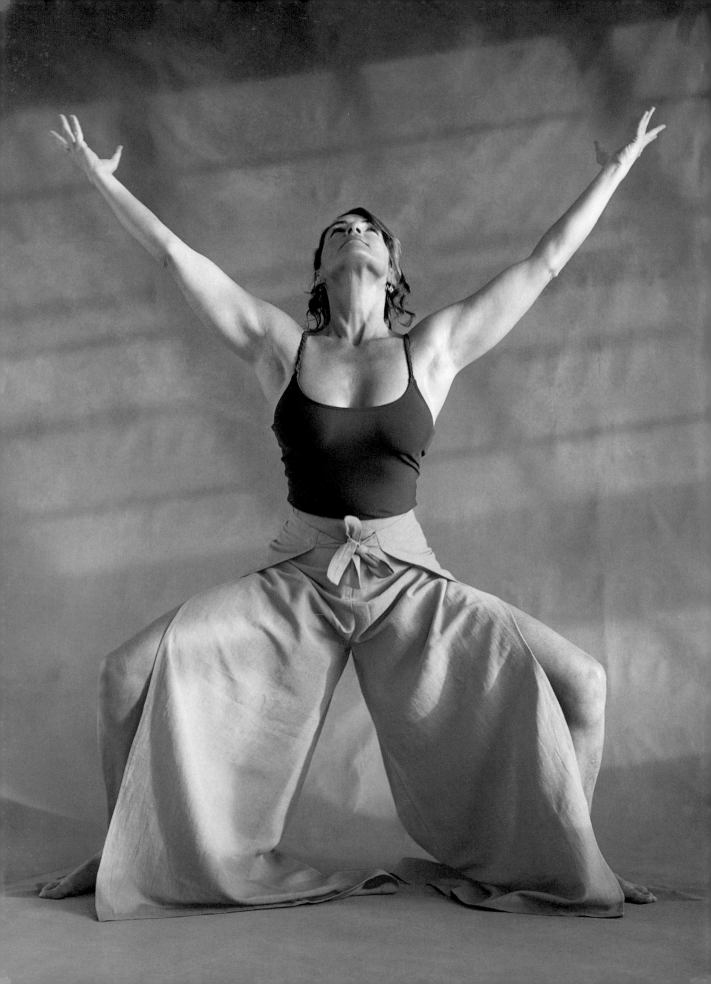

yoga and healing

The evolutionary history of humans is, and always has been, under threat from the forces of disease and environmental pressures. Apart from the continuing abuse of our planet's ecology with chemical pollution, we are still fighting each other on a terrifying scale. Military confrontations seem to be a manifestation of cultural, political and economic rivalries, reflecting part of the value system dominant in our society: one that emphasizes competition over cooperation.

And although we live in a time of awe-inspiring progress in science, facilitated to a large extent by technological innovation, we continue to suffer from large-scale infections and diseases that sweep societies and which have no political or geographical boundaries. Our advances in technology are only as good as their applications. Modern medicine is characterized by the wide scale use of pharmaceutical drugs, the product of huge financial investment and bio-chemical technology. Drug therapy has become so commonplace that it is often the mainstay of treatment by the medical profession. Alternative methods of treatment – for high blood pressure, for example – are rarely considered, with the result that a patient is often left dependant on a synthetic drug for life, a situation not without drawbacks. Synthetic drugs have, of course, saved many lives and increased life expectancy. However, our conditioning to run to the doctor at the slightest sign of a cold or headache have overburdened our human resources and fuelled the growth of the pharmaceutical industry.

Our modern day 'quick-fix' culture has tended to encourage an external projection of blame for our illnesses and complaints, rather than self-analysis and introspection; a 'cure' from without rather than from within. If we can nurture the motivation and courage to take some responsibility for our own health, we may surprise ourselves with the benefits that can be reaped.

To help oneself it is useful to first have a basic understanding of the problem with which one is dealing, in whatever context that may be. For the average lay person, the field of health, disease and medicine is clouded in mystery, partly due to the complexity of the language employed and partly due to time constraints on doctors, limiting them in their role as educators.

The aim of this book is not to contradict the prescription of what may be essential medication, but to empower the average person to understand more about the workings of their own body, the concept of health and the causes of disease so, where possible, they can help themselves. Yoga, often misunderstood to be either purely exercise or purely meditation, can be a powerful method of self-healing for the mind as well as the body. Even when we are in a healthy state, the application of yoga philosophies, principles and practices can have significant effects on our wellbeing. The effects can, however, be all the more profound when we are in a state of disorder or 'dis-ease'.

East–West Practices

To appreciate our contemporary approach and our methods used in dealing with disease, it is helpful to have a broader historical perspective on medical theories and practices. Ancient cultures the world over, whether Aztecs, Incas, Chinese, Indian, Egyptian, Greek or Roman, recognized the inherently multidimensional nature of health and disease. In general, they viewed disease as the dissociation and fragmentation of nature and spirit and therefore used an eclectic range of modalities to maintain, enhance and restore health. Their emphasis may have varied from association with deities or the spirit world to more basic considerations of the person and their interaction with the environment, but the common theme was one of recognition of health and disease states as being multifactorial – influenced by a variety of both internal as well as external factors.

Traditional medical systems are theoretical, practical systems developed by the major civilizations of the world, which have been documented and passed on in written texts for thousands of years. Broadly categorized into Western and Eastern systems, the main Eastern systems are traditional Chinese medicine and Ayurvedic medicine, an Indian system. The Western system, the root of modern medical science, can be traced back to what is popularly known as Hippocratic medicine.

SHAMANISM

According to shaministic traditions, human beings were viewed as part of a macrocosm, of which the spirit world was an integral part. Illness was therefore seen as a manifestation of a cosmic or moral disharmony. The restoration of harmony and balance between patient, nature and the spirit world was the primary objective of the shaman, a person able to voluntarily enter into an altered state of consciousness to make contact with the spirit world on behalf of their community. Shamans performed their duty with the help of certain hallucinogenic plants, the use of sounds such as drumming and chanting, and meditation. Therapeutic techniques included hypnosis, imagery, suggestion and dream analysis. This often took the form of a ritual with prayer and invocation, perhaps including the whole village so as to include a sociocultural element in the healing process. Helping a sick person was a common reason for such a practice, although it was also used to seek help regarding future decisions central to village life.

Shamans were therefore highly regarded and valued in their role as doctor, spiritual leader and often village chief. Because basic medical knowledge was passed on experientially among the community, the intervention of the shaman was only required in special cases … a very different case from our modern-day doctor!

THE HIPPOCRATIC TRADITION

The ancient Greeks regarded healing as primarily a spiritual phenomenon, represented by certain deities in mythology. The goddess Hygieia's name meant 'health', a term used to represent the preventative dimension of heeding nature's laws. Her sister was Panakeia, meaning 'all-healing' and representing the curative aspect of healing, derived from remedies in plants and in the earth. The search for a panacea has been a research priority of modern medical science, often at the expense of preventative health care and education.

Following a series of invasions and social changes around 2,000 BC, a male god Asclepius, hailed as father of the two daughters and the dominant healing god, was worshipped. A ritual form of 'asclepian' healing involved dream analysis during temple incubation, which reflected the Greek's belief in the god's healing power. The cult of Asclepius was symbolized by a serpent coiling around the Asclepian staff and has endured through history as the symbol of Western medicine.

Around that time a physician, highly skilled in the use of remedies and surgery, is said to have existed by the same name and was credited as the founder of medicine. Out of this mortal tradition grew the pinnacle of Greek medical knowledge – the *Hippocratic Corpus*. This huge collection of medical writings is attributed to a famous Asclepian physician known as Hippocrates, living around 400 BC on the island of Cos, although the text is probably the result of combined input from various Asclepian guilds and, significantly, Egyptian sources.

The Hippocratic tradition was concerned with the prevention of illnesses but also endeavoured to follow a scientific method of diagnosis and therapy. Health was viewed as a state of balance and included the influence of the environment and lifestyle on both physical and psycho-emotional factors. The physical elements were known as 'humours', referring to the biochemical aspects of the body; the psycho-emotional ones were known as 'passions', relating to both mental health and the mind/body connection. Hippocrates recognized that the healing power of nature pervaded all living organisms and saw the role of the physician as simply assisting this process by creating the optimum conditions for self-healing. This same philosophy remains the fundamental concept in modern-day naturopathy.

TRADITIONAL CHINESE MEDICINE

In the East, classical Chinese medicine was formalized and documented between 206 BC to 220 AD in various texts, the most important text being the *Nei Ching*, which contains theories of both medicine and the human organism in health and disease. The practice can be seen as an extension of Taoism, which recognizes the cyclical nature of the universe with all things in it affected – the macrocosm affecting the microcosm and vice versa. Human beings are seen in relation to and affected by cosmology, the seasons, diurnal cycles and times of day. Quality of sleep, food and emotional states were considered important factors influencing overall health.

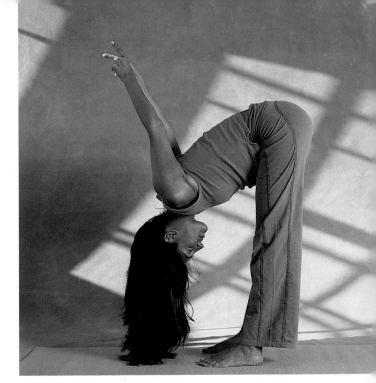

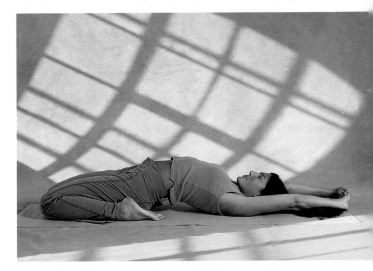

TOP TO BOTTOM **Makko-Ho stretches, from the Chinese medical tradition, balance the six meridians in the body (see page 10). The standing forward bend, padottanasana, top, attends to the lungs and large intestine (metal energy). It is linked to grief, breathing, vitality and dryness. The reclining hero pose, supta virasana, shown centre, relates to the stomach and spleen (earth energy) and meridians in the chest, throat, knees, shins and feet. It is linked to intellect, digestion, the flesh and blood. The butterfly, baddha konasana, bottom, attends to the heart and small intestine (fire energy). It is linked to the complexion, sweating, circulation, emotional repression and joy.**

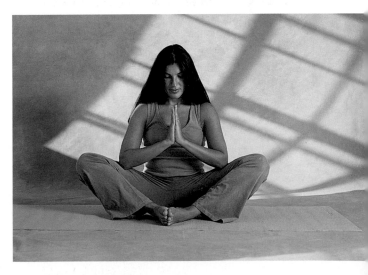

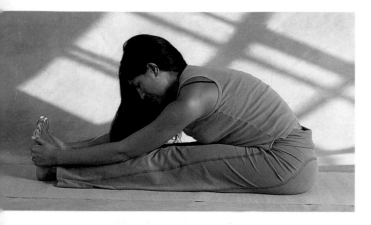

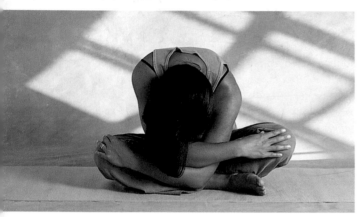

TOP TO BOTTOM The seated bend, pachimottanasana, top, relates to the kidneys and bladder (water energy). It is linked to will power, fear, fatigue, reproduction, growth and bones. The crossed-leg position, above, is a heart protector (fire energy) and linked to emotional defence, circulation, infection and allergies. Related to the liver and gall bladder (wood energy), the side bend, upavistha konasana, below, is linked to muscle stiffness and uneven emotions.

As regards the body itself, the Chinese stressed the importance of function and inter-relations of body parts, which is reflected in the meridian model. According to Chinese medicine, meridians are pathways of energy (or 'chi') in the body, and there are six pairs, each relating to a different body part. Harmonizing the flow of these pathways can restore and rebalance organ function, and Makko-Ho stretches can be employed to balance each one (see page 9 and left). Chinese medicine also employs the philosophical concepts of yin and yang, the archetypal polar opposites between which the various components of the universe fluctuate. The Chinese medical model is further complicated by the Wu Hsing, commonly translated as 'the five elements' – wood, fire, earth, metal and water. The five elements are seen to either give rise to each other or conquer each other. As such, they are a metaphysical explanation of the progression of change that can be applied to everything one encounters in the world – from politics to weather to biology. By using this paradigm of cyclical patterns and energy flow, the workings of the human body are explained within the context of the universe as a whole.

AYURVEDIC PRINCIPLES

The Indian medical system of Ayurveda – meaning the 'science of life' – has a similar pedigree to that of traditional Chinese medicine, dating back to an original text, the *Caraka Samhita*, written around 200–300 BC. The Ayurvedic view of health and disease is similarly wide in scope, seeing the human being as an integral part of nature and the universe. It recognizes three principles in nature known as gunas, namely energy or drive (rajas), inertia (tamas) and light (sattwa). These are seen to impart qualities that influence our mental state. In addition there are five elements, called panchamahabhutas, that differ slightly from the Chinese

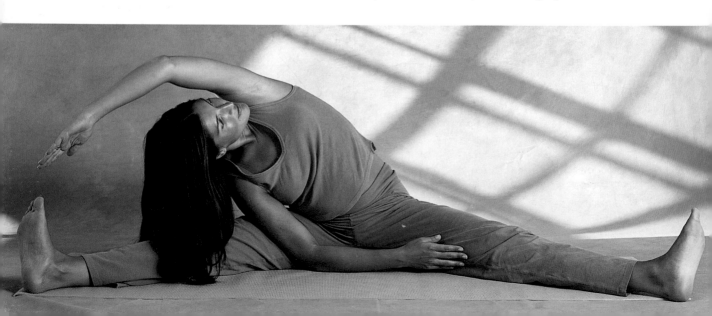

model. They are, in a hierarchical order from gross to subtle: earth, water, fire, air and space. Their properties can be seen to impart qualities to our bodies depending on their combination in each individual.

The inherent dynamic tendency for our bodies to fluctuate along the health/disease continuum is recognized by the Ayurvedic concept of doshas – known as pitta, vata and kapha – which are unstable qualities that control all the functions of the body. The derivation of the term doshas comes from *dus*, meaning 'to become spoiled', alluding to our physiological susceptibility to harmful foods, emotional states and so on. Pitta is responsible for heat and metabolism, vata for motion and rhythm of life, and kapha is the stabilizing force responsible for growth and cohesion. According to Ayurvedic thought, our constitution is a product of the balance of the doshas inherited through the semen and ovum (now known as genetic inheritance), with a balance of all three doshas being the most desirable.

When the doshas are out of balance, they also disturb other body tissues (dhatus) and functions such as the elimination of waste (malas). Thus, the criteria for health from the Ayurvedic perspective is when the doshas are in equilibrium, the digestive 'fire' (called agni) is balanced, the body tissues/wastes are in the right amount and proportion, and the senses, mind and soul are content. Although yoga is recognized as the sister of Ayurveda, yoga practices can be seen as a form of medicine in their own right. Traditional Chinese medicine also uses physical exercise, such as chi kung and tai chi, as a complement to therapy.

The Yoga Treatment

Derived from the old English word 'whole', 'holy' or 'complete', the word 'healing' implies a journey towards wholeness, and health is an ever-changing state wherein the various systems within the body maintain a complex inter-relationship of dynamic harmony. Dr Vasant Lad, author of *Ayurveda: The Science of Self-Healing*, describes health as order and disease as disorder, explaining that disease occurs when the internal body is 'out of synch' with its external surroundings. Yogic practices offer the potential for us to gain control over our apparently unconscious internal workings and become our own healers. This necessitates cultivating sensitivity in order to detect when imbalance occurs. Sometimes being laid out flat on our back is the only way that nature can show us how to restore ourselves, and illness can be viewed as a wake-up call when we are complacent. While modern medicine concentrates on the apparent manifestation of the material (the body), yoga medicine focuses on the subtle infrastructure – the invisible essence within that container: bioenergy, or prana (see page 12).

Yoga techniques seek to uproot negative patterns and expand the potent forces of the mind – through the vehicle of the body and breath – to restore equilibrium. In the following chapters, asanas (postures), pranayamas (breathing practices), yoga nidra (deep relaxation), along with meditations and 'cleansings' are prescribed.

ASANA SEQUENCES – VINYASAS

Sequences of postures are presented in this book to suit all levels. Always adapt to your ability and never strain. The order in which postures are sequenced is called vinyasa ('to place in a special way'), and can change mood, breathing pattern, nervous system functioning, hormonal balance and blood pressure, as well as your internal organic behaviour. Most postures, apart from elongations, end with counterposes (pratikriya), which create an opposite action to the one preceding, making each sequence safe and complete. The way in which we practise yoga has tremendous impact: long holds and inversions are particularly healing, drawing the blood back towards the centre of the body from the extremities and activating parasympathetic nervous activity. Calming postures, such as forward bends, twists and inversions, facilitate healing, while energizing postures, such as laterals and backbends, are more uplifting.

Forward bends are embryonic and soothing, encouraging introspection. They nourish digestive and reproductive systems, and calm the adrenals.

Backbends are energizing and uplifting, as they unfold and open the body, and encourage extroversion. They nourish the digestive, respiratory and circulatory systems, and balance the thymus, adrenal and thyroid glands.

Lateral stretches are energizing and aligning. They nourish circulatory and respiratory systems, and soothe the adrenals.

Twists are calming and integrating, as they balance introversion and extroversion, the right and left sides of the body and brain, and logic and intuition. They nourish the digestive system and balance the adrenal, gonad and thyroid glands.

Extensions balance activity of the front and back body. They nourish the reproductive and digestive systems, and balance the gonads (organs that produce sex cells).

Inversions are restorative and soothing. They nourish the circulatory system and remove strain from the body and mind. In addition, they balance the pineal, pituitary and thyroid glands.

The Language of the Body

'HEALING MAY NOT BE SO MUCH ABOUT
GETTING BETTER AS ABOUT LETTING GO OF
EVERYTHING THAT ISN'T YOU – ALL OF THE
EXPECTATIONS, ALL OF THE BELIEFS – AND
BECOMING WHO YOU ARE. NOT A BETTER
YOU, BUT A REALER YOU.'

Dr Remen, *The Human Patient*

The yogic concept of the body is of a multilayered
jacket made up of five sheaths – koshas – each finer
and more subtle as you travel to the interior. The
outer is called annamaya kosha, the physical
body; pranamayakosha is the energy body; the
manomayakosah is the mental body (lower mind);
vijnanamayakosha is the psychic body (higher mind); and
the innermost sheath is called anandamayakosha, the
bliss body. Each layer is nourished by the layer beneath
it. If we do not nourish the subtle inner layer, the body's
outer manifestation may be disordered or unharmonious.

PRANA: THE LIFE FORCE

Described as bioenergy, prana is the all-pervading
essence which organizes, activates and animates all the
koshas, including the physical body. Channelled through
tiny streams in the subtle body called 'nadis', prana is
cultivated through pranayama (breathing techniques),
which control psychic and vital energy. Considered to
bridge the mind with the body, clear-flowing prana
awakens somatic intelligence and, with thought-power
and visualization, can be directed as a healing force.

Prana manifests in five patterns – vayus – in the body.
Concerned with hunger and thirst, prana is the vitalizing,
internalizing force centred around the chest, heart and
head. It is expansive, spreading and associated with fire.
Apana, its opposite, is the descending energy, focused
in the physical body below the navel. It is a rooting,
downward pattern of expulsion, throwing out impurities
through elimination of faeces, urine and ejaculation.
Apana is also the force of childbirth. Located at the root
chakra, it is grounding and stabilizing. It aids movement
through the intestines and relates to the element of earth.
These two primary forces – ascending and descending –
are constantly at play throughout yoga practice.

In addition to prana and apana, there are three more
patterns within the microcosm of the body, each relating
to particular functions and elements. Samana is centring,
assimilating energy, which activates and controls
digestion. Associated with the stomach, liver, pancreas
and small intestine, its balancing energy is centred at the

navel. It is concerned with the secretion of juices and
assimilation of nutrients, preparing the essence (rasa) of
food and distributing the rasa to the relevant places in the
body via the blood river. Samana relates to the element
water. Udana is the ascending energy, sited at the throat
and above in the physical body, the energy that keeps the
body 'on its toes', upright. Connected to the processes
of belching and vomiting, it is associated with the element
air. Finally, vyana is an expanding energy, which pervades
the whole body. It is concerned with the distributive force
that performs all the bodily functions, particularly heart
and limbs, and keeps the sensory nerves active. Vyana
is also associated with ether (space).

NADIS

The pathways of prana run like sap through tiny streams
called nadis in the body, numbering 72,000, though we
are concerned with three: the trunk and its tributaries.

The essential prana is channelled through sushumna
nadi, which flows through the centre of the spinal cord
and is associated with the central nervous system, the
central highway to the brain. Weaving around the central
channel run two snakelike channels in a knot formation,
which originate from their source at the muladhara
chakra (see chakras, pages 14–15). Ida, the moon
channel, originates from the left side of muladhara
chakra at the perineum. A cool, passive energy, it
represents the parasympathetic nervous system and
relates to venous blood in the circulatory system. It is
dominant when the breath is flowing through the left
nostril. Pingala, the sun channel, originates from the right
side of muladhara chakra and is a dynamic, extrovert
and active energy. It represents the sympathetic nervous
system and relates to the flow of arterial blood in the
circulatory system, dominant when the breath is flowing
through the right nostril (see nadi shodana, page 121).

In our driven culture, many of us function
predominantly on sympathetic or nervous activity (see
also pages 35–37), wherein we are continually charged
to the point where we do not know how to 'clock off'.
The primary aim of Hatha yoga ('Ha' meaning sun and
denoting ambition and 'tha' meaning moon and implying
restoration) is to merge the two energies into the central
channel of sushumna (see above), in order to attain yogic
oneness. Yoga is concerned with dissolving duality and
this is explored in yoga practice when we seek to draw
prana and apana together.

OPPOSITE **This pose symbolizes the creative spiral of
the kundalini serpent – the metaphor given to one's latent
energy that lies locked in a coil in the sacrum, below the
navel. Yoga practices aim to access this internal energy.**

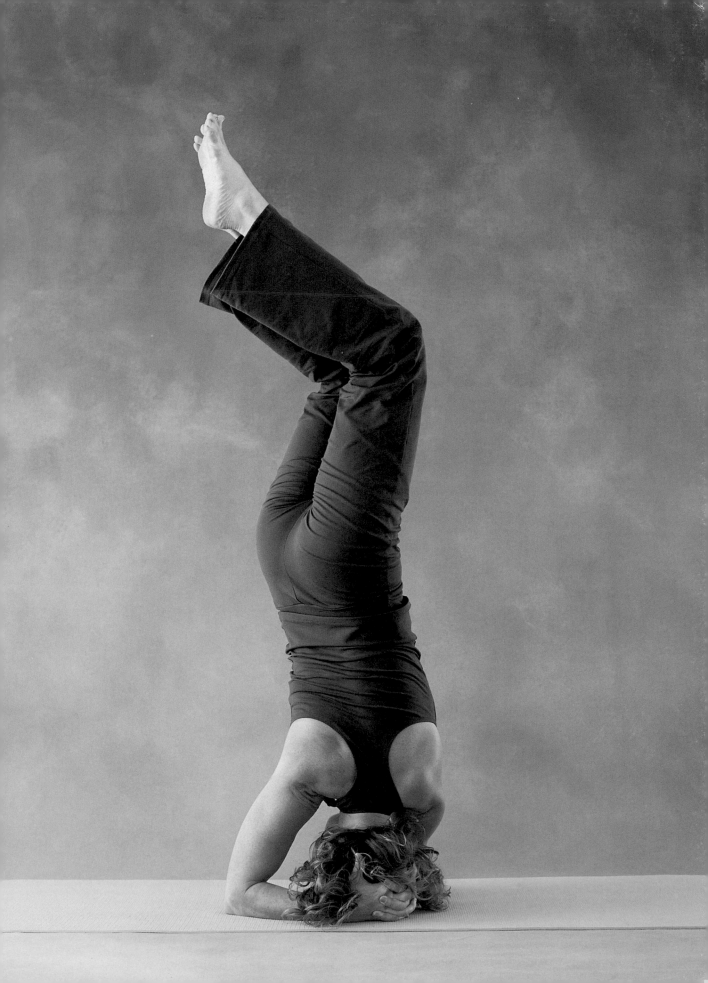

CHAKRAS

The chakra model can be viewed as a symbolic study of the human system, a subtle map to chart the multidimensional aspects of the human being. Described as whirling vortexes of energy, represented as lotus flowers, seven chakras spin at different junctions along the axis of the spinal stem. Each corresponds with nerve plexi, endocrine glands and vital organs.

Associated with an element, seed syllable (bija mantra) and visual representation (yantra), each chakra forms an archetypal framework to study the Self, located at psychosomatic points. Esoteric, yet embedded in the tangible fabric of the body, meditations on the chakras and their corresponding attributes can offer much in understanding, integrating and resonating with our lives.

Organized around sushumna nadi, the central energy channel through the spinal stem, chakras spin at junctions, where the three major nadis converge in their ascending weave. Each chakra is said to have 18 attributes, and here we look at several of these.

BELOW, LEFT TO RIGHT **These pictures are a contemporary interpretation of the chakras, based on classical Indian Dance. Yoga and Indian Dance are synonymous, each cultivating rasa, the essence of ultimate enjoyment, and linking the mind and body. The connection is embodied in this sloka, or Sanskrit text, from the second century AD:**

> *Where the hand goes, the eyes follow,*
> *Where the eyes go, mind follows,*
> *Where the mind goes, there feelings are cultivated;*
> *Where there are feelings, there is enjoyment.*

MULADHARA, THE EARTH ELEMENT

The 'root support' chakra is the psychic centre located at the perineum, corresponding from the hips to the feet, connecting one to basic survival, primitive instincts and security. This foundation lock at the floor (or door) of the torso is the seat of sexual and spiritual energy and represents physical, mental and emotional stability. If this root is not secure, we flounder, looking outside for stability rather than cultivating our own inner ground.

❀ **Nerve plexus:** sacrococcygeal
❀ **Associated organs/glands:** perineum/pelvic diaphragm
❀ **Colour:** red
❀ **Yantra:** red square
❀ **Mantra:** Lam
❀ **Affirmation:** 'I trust. I am secure.' 'My home is within me.'

SWADHISTANA, THE WATER ELEMENT

Located at the level of the pubic bone, the frontal bone of the pelvis (the body's centre of gravity and the seat of feeling), swadhistana translates as 'self-sustaining' and is connected to pleasure, creativity and relationships. Housed in the sacrum, it is linked to sexuality and socialization, and organically related to the genitals, the bladder and kidneys (water).

❀ **Nerve plexus:** sacrococcygeal
❀ **Associated organs/glands:** reproductive organs
❀ **Colour:** orange
❀ **Yantra:** upward-facing crescent moon
❀ **Mantra:** Vam
❀ **Affirmation:** 'Pantha Rei.' 'Flow like water.' 'I yield.'

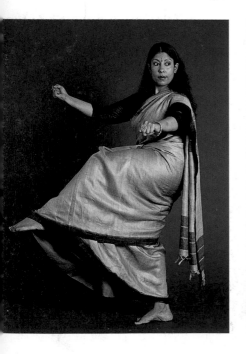 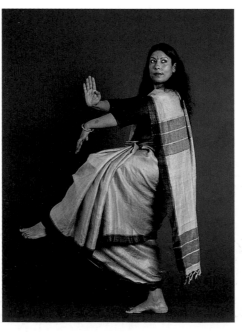 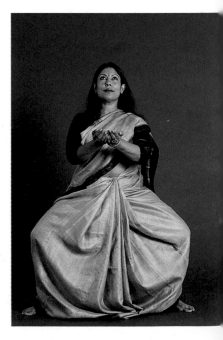

MANIPURA, THE FIRE ELEMENT

Situated at the solar plexus, manipura is associated with vitality, drive, self-esteem and energy, translating as 'city of gems'. The seat of agni, it represents ambition and transformation, digestion being an expression of this.

* **Nerve plexus:** solar plexus
* **Associated organs/glands:** digestive organs
* **Colour:** yellow
* **Yantra:** triangle
* **Mantra:** Ram
* **Affirmation:** 'I digest all experiences.'

ANAHATA, THE AIR ELEMENT

The root of emotions, situated behind the breastbone at the base of the sternum, anahata relates to the thoracic spine, heart, lungs and spleen. This chakra is the gateway from the earthbound to the transcendent. It relates to giving, receiving, devotion and surrender.

* **Nerve plexus:** cardiac plexus
* **Associated organs/glands:** thymus/heart
* **Colour:** green
* **Yantra:** hexagon
* **Mantra:** Yam
* **Affirmation:** 'My vulnerability is my strength.'

VISHUDDHI, THE SPACE ELEMENT

Sited behind the throat, vishuddhi means 'extraordinarily pure', and relates to the cervical spine, thymus and thyroid glands, throat and voice. It is linked with sound and hearing, instruments of expression which require an awareness of space in order to communicate artfully.

* **Nerve plexus:** laryngeal
* **Associated organs/glands:** thyroid
* **Colour:** turquoise
* **Yantra:** circle
* **Mantra:** Ham
* **Affirmation:** 'Clarity sustains me.' 'I see uncoloured.'

AJNA, THE HIGHER INTELLIGENCE

The seat of intuition, situated in the midbrain, ajna means 'all knowing', signifying discernment and discrimination. The 'third eye' awareness is embodied here, leading to freedom from attachments that cause suffering.

* **Associated organs/glands:** pineal
* **Colour:** magenta
* **Yantra:** often depicted as an upward-pointing crescent moon above a downward-pointing triangle
* **Mantra:** Om
* **Affirmation:** 'I perceive with my wisdom mind.'

SAHASRARA, THE THOUSAND SPOKES

At the crown of the head, this chakra embodies transcendent awareness and higher consciousness. It represents the fully integrated human being, a state wherein all the chakras are vibrantly spinning, alive in every cell. In yoga this is called samadhi, a state where all boundaries are dissolved and oneness occurs.

* **Associated organs/glands:** pituitary
* **Colour:** purple
* **Yantra:** often represented by a full, moon-like circle
* **Mantra:** Om
* **Affirmation:** 'I and the Source are One.'

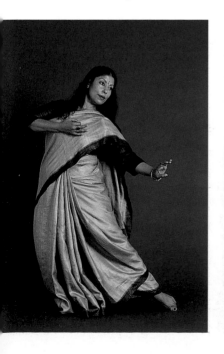
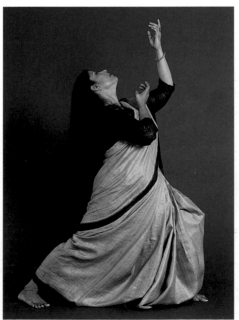
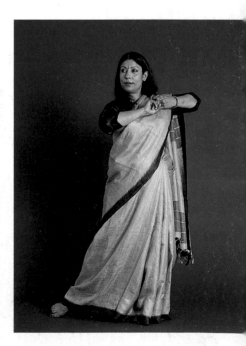

BANDHAS

The most common translation of the word 'bandha' is 'lock' or 'seal', which helps to explain their function on a physical level. Bandhas are traditionally prescribed as a tool for 'untying' the psychic 'knots' or granthis in the chakras. This is also a paradox: on the psychic level, bandhas are seen as tools for 'unlocking' blockages within the chakras and along the upward path of the sushumna nadi. The bandhas are essentially a physical contraction of certain muscles which exert widespread affects on neurological, circulatory, respiratory and endocrine function with associated emotional and psychic ramifications. There are three primary bandhas: mula, uddiyana and jalandhara bandha, involving contraction of the perineal (pelvic), abdominal and cervical (neck) muscles respectively. When contracted simultaneously, this is called maha bandha, the 'great seal'.

MULA BANDHA

The words 'mula' and 'bandha' refer to the contraction of muladhara chakra, the seat of kundalini (see page 14). The attention given to this practice is due to the belief that the stimulation of muladhara chakra will begin the process of awakening this energy for the journey to transcendental consciousness. The energy of this psychic centre is thought to be accessed on a physical level by the contraction of the perineal body in the male and the cervix in women.

The complexity of the anatomy and the correct use of terminology need to be understood to appreciate the subtlety of mula bandha. The anatomical perineum is a diamond-shaped region commonly referred to as the 'pelvic floor' – the sling of muscles around the sphincters of the urethra, vagina and anus known as the pubo-coccygeus. This is distinct from the more discreet structure of the perineal body used in mula bandha (see also page 89). It is the perineal body that is usually implied by yoga teachers when asking students to contract their perineum. Mula bandha may be confused with other forms of pelvic floor contraction which are also yogic techniques, such as ashwini mudra, the much grosser action of contracting the gluteals, anal sphincter and pelvic diaphragm, and vajroli mudra, which is a contraction of the urogenital muscles (see pages 88–89).

Initially, most people will contract the anal sphincter to engage the perineum until the awareness improves to differentiate the various components of the pelvic floor – namely, the anal sphincter, the urogenital muscles and the pelvic diaphragm. Performed correctly, mula bandha is a gentle contraction of the urogenital muscles and the pelvic diaphragm.

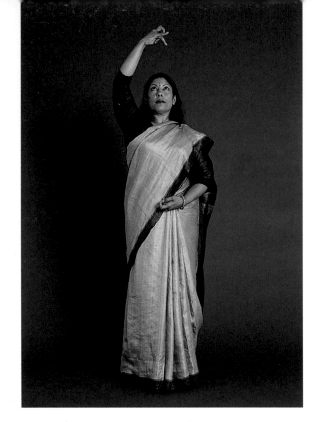

ABOVE **This is an interpretation of the vertical axis of the spine. When all chakras are resonating, divine alignment occurs and one is in a state of yogic union.**

An easy method of creating the gross sensation of mula bandha is to perform a mock exhalation (keeping the mouth closed) as if bearing down to go to the toilet but also resisting that pressure with the whole pelvic floor as well as the abdominal wall. This manoeuvre should have enlisted resistance from the muscles of the pelvic diaphragm and urogenital muscles without significant activity of the anal sphincter. Breathing out slowly but deeply while drawing the abdominal wall in towards the spine should elicit a mild squeezing of the area between the anus and genitals. This exercise will begin to cultivate the sensation of mula bandha, which becomes less natural when the balance point is rocked back towards the coccyx as in a slumped sitting posture, in which case the emphasis shifts towards the anal triangle/anal sphincter.

The effects of mula bandha are profound and widespread, and the practice is revered by yogis as a pranic rather than a physical technique. It maintains a healthy pelvic floor and cultivates a sensation of lightness and wellbeing. Mula bandha helps to contain intra-abdominal pressure thereby encouraging healthy circulation within the abdomino-pelvic cavity, in turn promoting heathy organ function. It should not be practised if you suffer from heart problems, high blood pressure, high intracranial pressure, vertigo or amenorrhea (unnatural cessation of menstruation).

UDDIYANA BANDHA

Called the flying-up lock, uddiyana bandha is a yogic exercise that involves suction of the abdominal wall towards the spine following a full exhalation. It should be practised on an empty stomach. The action compresses the abdominal organs and also the solar plexus.

To perform, stand with the knees slightly bent and the hands resting on the thighs just above the knees to transfer bodyweight away from the trunk muscles and position the abdominal organs forwards in the abdominal cavity. Exhale maximally, then perform a mock inhalation with the rib cage by closing the glottis (top of the airway) to prevent any influx of air. The application of jalandhara bandha (see below) helps to create a stable base to reinforce the action of closing the glottis. Keeping the abdomen relaxed while still holding the breath, further suck up the abdominal wall so that the abdomen becomes concave underneath the rib cage. Mula bandha (see opposite) can be consciously engaged at the same time, although this feeling will probably happen naturally.

Maintain for a few seconds but be careful not to overstrain. Stop if any lightheadedness is experienced. To exit, first reduce the vacuum in the thorax by slowly releasing the suction of the abdominal wall to allow the diaphragm and abdominal organs to descend and abdomino/thoracic pressures to stabilize. Just before breathing in, compress the abdomen/chest again to return lung/atmospheric pressures to their normal ratios, otherwise air will be sucked in due to a lowered thoracic pressure.

Uddiyana banda tones the muscles of the abdominal wall and stretches the vertically orientated muscle fibres of the diaphragm. It reduces the 'drag' effect of gravity on the abdominal contents by lifting them upwards within the abdominal cavity. Caution: Do not practise it if you suffer from high blood pressure, high intracranial pressure, glaucoma, ulcers, ulcerative colitis, hiatus hernia, or during pregnancy or menstruation.

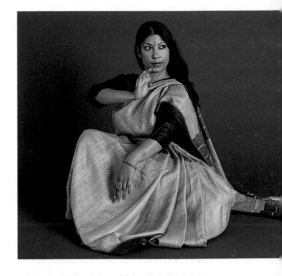

JALANDHARA BANDHA

This bandha is the 'chin lock', which can be created voluntarily or may naturally occur due to the nature of an asana (for example, the plough, halasana). It involves the action of drawing the chin back and down towards the supra-sternal notch. To varying degrees, depending upon asana, jalandhara bandha compresses the carotid sinus and has the reflex effect of reducing the heart rate and blood pressure. It narrows the airway at the glottis, helping to slow down or regulate the breath, which is particularly beneficial in inverted or meditative asanas. Jalandhara bandha lengthens the muscles of the back of the neck, and filters air and extracts prana. Caution: Avoid it, or asanas that place the body naturally in jalandhara, if you suffer from neck problems, respiratory disorders (particularly if a panic breath is provoked), high blood pressure, intra-cranial pressure or coronary heart disease.

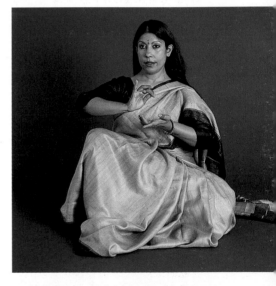

TOP TO BOTTOM **Physical gesturing as a ritualistic practice – using the hands, eyes and even the whole body as a symbolic prayer – has been used in all major religions. The medieval Dominican Order of the Friars practised genuflections and gestures; Islamic prayers involve whole-body movements; and yogasanas and sun salutations demonstrate the body as an alchemical vessel for the spirit. Hand gestures subtly attune the mind and can be practised while performing mantras or pranayamas.**

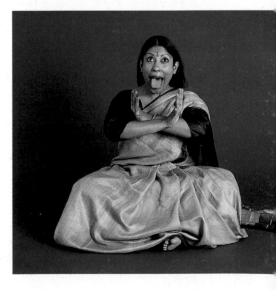

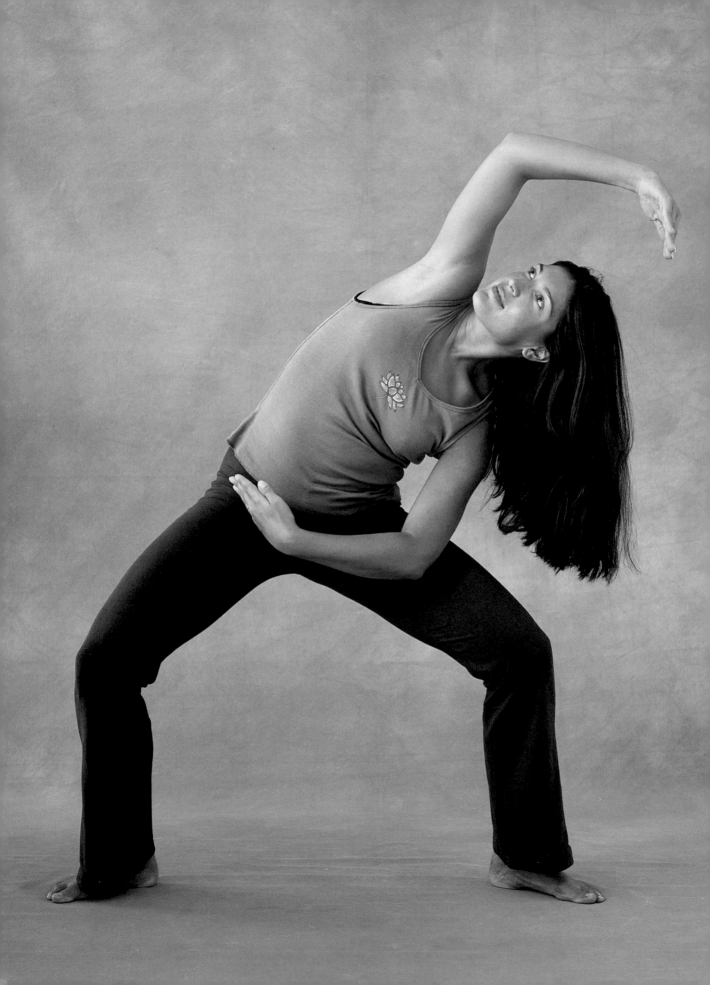

the respiratory system:

breathing the yoga way

The breath is the tide of life, nourishing us into eternity, and breathing rhythms affect our state of consciousness. The yogic view is that the breath is a direct mirror of the quality of the mind, and irregular or incorrect breathing reflects a scattered mind and a lack of the mind/body connection. As such, breath is indicative of health, and chaotic breathing eventually manifests itself as disease. Learning to breathe freely, observing the breath so that it gradually penetrates every cell of our body, is therefore fundamental to healing.

Physical, mental and emotional stress impress upon on the way we breathe and, likewise, the way we breathe can affect our psychophysiology. The breath contains thoughtwaves, which can be unravelled. In yoga we aim to repattern the breath gently, unravelling its threads to gradually dislodge habitual 'holding' patterns reflecting mental tension. According to Dr Alexander Lowen's school of bioenergy, abnormal breathing is a sign of inhibited feelings, such as anger or resentment, which may contribute to disorders including asthmatic attacks and habitual muscular tension combined with inhibited breathing reflecting underlying disharmony. The practice of pranayamas restores the balance of the inbreath and the outbreath. The inbreath is energizing, expansive and creative; the outbreath calming, centring and rooting. An expansive inbreath is called 'brahmana' (solar) breath; a deep outbreath is called 'langhana' (lunar) breath.

THE RESPIRATORY SYSTEM

Respiration is more than just breathing. It is divided into two types: internal respiration is the diffusion of gases, mainly oxygen and carbon dioxide, across the capillary walls and tissue cell membranes whereas external respiration is the diffusion of the same gases across the capillary walls and alveoli (tiny air sacs of the lungs). Both rely on the cardiovascular system for efficient function. The upper respiratory tract includes the sinuses, nose, mouth and pharynx; the lower respiratory tract includes the larynx, trachea, bronchi and lungs.

ABDOMINAL AND CHEST BREATHING

Poor health can be the result of the mechanism of breathing used – chest or abdominal breathing – or by the characteristics of the inhale/exhale relationship. Abdominal breathing, sometimes termed 'diaphragmatic' breathing, is used here to describe the pattern of predominantly abdominal expansion on inhalation; chest or 'thoracic' breathing is used to describe the pattern of predominantly chest/rib expansion on inhalation.

Possible reasons for an inability to abdominal breathe fully may include:

- Habitual tension pattern of shallow breathing
- Emotional holding pattern in the abdomen
- History of lower back pain/disc problems creating guarding of the abdominal wall
- Contraction of the abdominal wall due to excessive amounts of abdominal exercises
- Difficulty exhaling, as in asthma 'wheezing', so that the abdominal muscles are habitually recruited for an active (forced) exhalation. This leads to chronic tightening of the abdominal wall.

Some individuals cannot fully expand their chest cavity. The possible reasons may include:

- Lack of aerobic exercise over a sustained period
- Smoking
- Trauma to upper back, ribs or sternum
- Congenital malformations of sternum or spine, such as scoliosis (lateral spinal curvature)
- Weak abdominal muscles, for example as a result of abdomino-pelvic surgery
- Chronic constipation or abdominal bloating, as in Irritable Bowel Syndrome (IBS)
- History of chronic lung disease
- Lack of confidence/power.

A healthy body should have equal access to either mode of breathing. However, when one mode becomes difficult, the other mode predominates by default and it is this inability to switch modes voluntarily that constitutes a 'breathing' imbalance. A general rule to follow may be to improve the function of whichever mode is deficient.

Abdominal breathing is the natural breathing method when the body is at rest, as it demands less effort physically. It is associated with relaxation and the parasympathetic nervous system.

Thoracic breathing is an energetic breath mostly associated with exercise, the 'flight/fight response', and the need to utilize the full potential of the lungs to deliver oxygen to the system. A sprinter, for example, would chest breathe out of necessity, but anyone chest breathing while watching TV would be a strange sight indeed! It is important to point out at this stage that chest breathing can be performed in a calm manner and does not mean an adrenaline rush is an inevitable response! The power and benefits of the thoracic breath are sometimes overshadowed by an emphasis on the relaxing abdominal breath.

The abdomen and thorax represent a pressurized container divided by a muscular shelf – the diaphragm – which basically works as a piston inside a cylinder, creating an alternating pressure system similar to the original steam engine. When thoracic movement has become restricted due to either mechanical (rib joints and spine) or organic (lung) disorder, the downwards movement of the diaphragm becomes vital and is emphasized. The abdominal wall therefore swells forward to accommodate the extra pressure exerted by the diaphragm in its attempt to expand the volume of the thoracic cavity in a vertical direction.

It is no surprise that in many respiratory disorders the abdomen is often distended (exceptions being asthma and emphysema) as a result of this mechanism. Even in the absence of any diagnosed lung disorder, many people remain totally unaware of a reduction in their capacity to breathe using the thorax because the subtle shifts in breathing patterns take a long time, usually years, to occur. The inability to expand the rib cage significantly may be one external sign of lowered vitality in the body as it represents a diminished capacity to inhale fully.

A distended abdomen has its own sequelae, such as congestion of blood in the abdomino-pelvic organs and strain on the lower back and often the neck. This is an example of the knock-on effect of dysfunction in one system affecting others.

The control of the abdominal wall during inhalation is the most potent natural method we have of maximizing the volume of the rib cage and hence enhancing lung function. In yogic terms, the drawing back, or 'hollowing', of the abdominal wall towards the spine is known as uddiyana bandha (upward flying lock) and is performed on an exhalation as a technique in its own right (see page 17).

COMMON RESPIRATORY DISORDERS

Asthma is a reversible obstructive airway disease resulting in episodic periods of coughing and wheezing due to spasm of the smooth muscle of the small bronchi/bronchioles accompanied by overproduction of mucus, which partially obstructs the airways. An asthma attack is characterized by a difficulty in exhaling. The most common form of asthma is an allergic response to certain irritants in the environment, such as the house dust mite, pollen and certain foods, the most common of these being dairy and wheat. Allergic asthma is also associated with eczema and hayfever. Other irritants, including environmental pollutants and smoking (either active or passive), can also trigger an asthma attack. This disease is is also associated with emotional stress.

Emphysema occurs when the alveolar walls lose their inherent elasticity and remain full of air during expiration so that difficulty exhaling is the most notable symptom. As damaged alveoli coalesce to form even larger but dysfunctional air sacs, the lungs become permanently inflated and create a barrel chest appearance to accommodate the enlarged lungs, which begin to form fibrous tissue. Diffusion of respiratory gases then becomes even more difficult. The most common cause is smoking, but environmental/industrial pollutants can also be triggers.

Bronchitis is an infection of the bronchi that causes inflammation of the mucous membranes and glands lining them. The key symptom is a cough producing a yellow/greenish sputum. Infections may be acute or chronic. The most common causes are cigarette smoking and environmental pollution.

Sinusitis is an infection of the sinuses, which is usually associated with a cold. A cold is caused when the body succumbs to a viral infection, usually following times of stress and thus lowered immune function. The most common symptoms are proliferation of mucus in the nose, throat, sinuses and lungs, resulting in varying degrees of sneezing and coughing.

THERAPIES AND TREATMENTS

Orthodox treatment includes bronchodilators, steroids, antibiotics, decongestants and anti-inflammatory agents. Phase in the yoga practices given in this chapter gradually in tandem with the prescribed drugs. Maintain your required dose and monitor the effects: this may lead to reducing drug dependency although this should only be done in consultation with a doctor.

Other lifestyle recommendations that may help with respiratory problems are:
- Avoid overeating, which restricts the lungs due to distension of the stomach and intestines
- Avoid mucus-producing foods, such as wheat and milk products, fried and processed foods
- Try to drink freshly squeezed fruit/vegetable juice to reduce mucus while providing high levels of nutrients. Plenty of water also helps to thin mucus
- After eating, wash your hands and face and sit in comfortably for ten to fifteen minutes or take a slow, relaxed walk in the fresh air to 'clear' the lungs and passageways
- A 24-hour juice/water fast on a rest day will help flush out toxins.

Washing the Respiratory Tract/ Nasal Douche (Jala neti)

Traditional hatha yoga purification practices called shatkarmas remove toxins and impurities from the system, which increase energy levels and boost health. The practices number six ('shat'), though not all are recommended in the West. The cleanses should be learned direct under the specific guidance of a guru/ teacher as most are highly specialized, though jala neti is introduced here as it clears the breathing passages in a natural way (see also kapalbhati on page 30).

Jala neti is an excellent practice to prevent colds and clear excess mucus. It involves a nasal douche using a slightly salty, lukewarm water solution, flushed gently through the nasal passages with the use of a little pot called a neti lota (or you can simply use a breakfast bowl and inhale water through both nostrils).

Dissolve one teaspoon of salt in a litre (2.1 pints) of lukewarm water and pour into the neti lota or a similar small vessel or teapot. As you lean to one side the spout of the pot is inserted into one nostril, and the saline solution is gently poured through until it flows out of the opposite nostril. While breathing through the mouth, the water should be allowed to flow through for about 20 seconds. Alternate sides.

Basic Vinyasa

A mindful practice suitable for beginners or those recovering from illness, this vinyasa concentrates on expanding and opening the chest area to stimulate lung performance. It can help alleviate irregular breathing, asthma, emphysema and bronchitis. Vinyasa means 'to place in a special way'. We call yoga sequences vinyasas as they carefully and progressively open up the body, integrating breath with movement coordination.

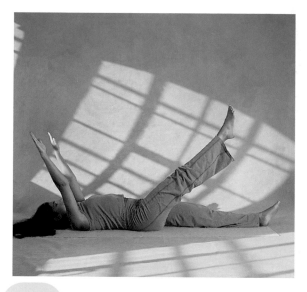

1 Lie flat with your arms resting alongside your body. Practise abdominal breathing into the lower belly. On inhale, raise the arms overhead until they reach the floor. On exhale, simultaneously lower the arms while raising the right leg.

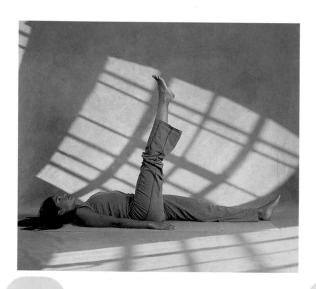

2 On the complete outbreath, lift the right leg to full vertical while pressing the palms down alongside you. Inhale, lower the right leg and raise the arms overhead. Now repeat with the left leg.

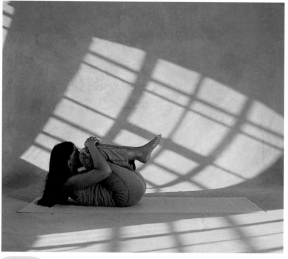

3 On exhale, lift the knees to the chest and raise the head, wrapping the arms around the shins. This is the knee-to-chest pose, apanasana. Hold and deepen the outbreath. On inhale, release your legs, relaxing your head and shoulders into the mat. Repeat three times.

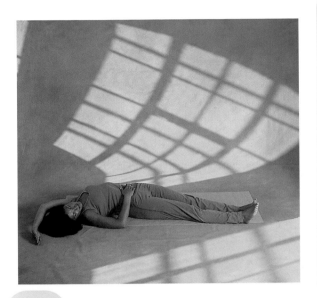

4 Lying supine, arc the body into a banana shape, with the head and feet to the right and hips to the left. Arch the left arm overhead and place the right hand on the belly. Practise the complete inhalation and exhalation, with awareness of the navel rising and falling, opening the left lung for ten breaths. Repeat on the other side.

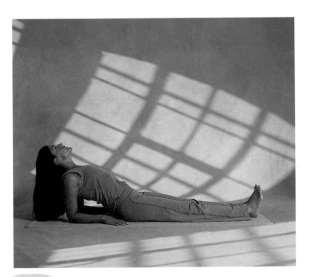

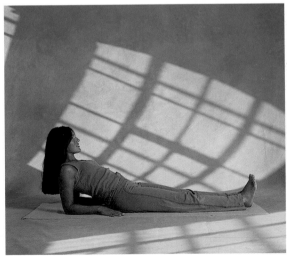

5 For expansion of the chest, practise the fish pose, matsyasana. Lie supine and on inhale, lift the upper torso to rest on the elbows, with the palms flat alongside the hips. Lift your chest high and carefully lower your head back with your chin to the sky.

On exhale, bring the chin forwards to the chest. On inhale, arch the spine and lift the chin to the sky; on exhale, bring the chin back to the chest. Repeat for five breaths. Now lie in the corpse pose (savasana) for some moments to observe the effects.

Intermediate Vinyasa, Sitting

The intermediate vinyasas stimulate the patterns of prana and apana (see page 12). They are particularly useful for sufferers of asthma, emphysema and bronchitis.

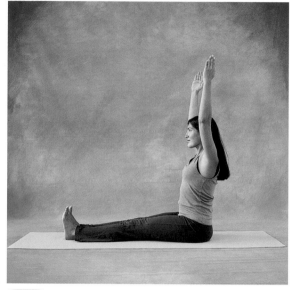

1 Sit with the legs straight and together, and arms by the sides. This is the staff pose, dandasana. Flex the feet and ground the sitting bones. Open the chest, lifting the sternum. On inhale, raise the arms above the head.

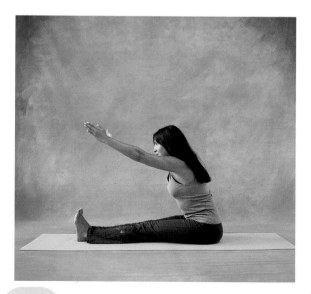

2 Exhale, draw the sternum forwards, pivoting at the hip joint into the seated forward bend, paschimottanasana. Breathe into the back ribs for ten breaths. Relax the shoulders away from the ears. Focus on exhalation as you deepen the bend.

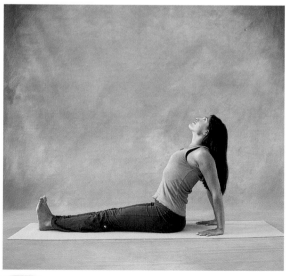

3 Inhale and return to seated, placing the palms flat about 30 cm (12 in) behind the hips, with the fingers pointing forwards. Roll the shoulders back, lifting the front armpits up. Exhale, press into the hands and point the toes.

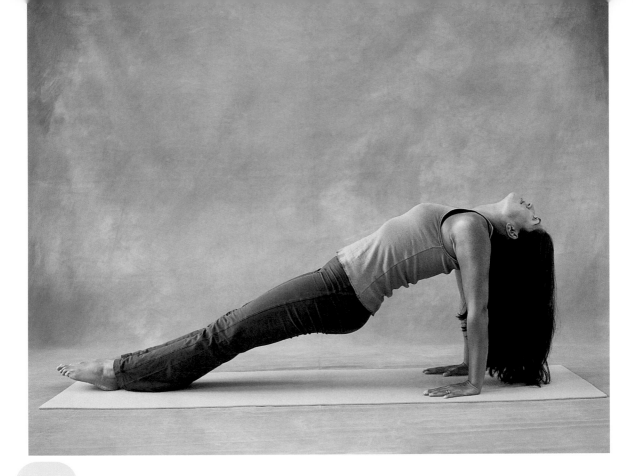

4 Inhale, lift the hips, coming into the plank pose, purvottanasana, stretching the front (east) of the body. Take five to ten breaths, depending on ability.

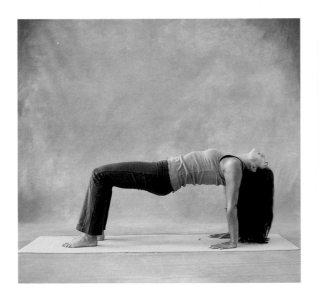

Modification: Alternatively, on inhale, lift into table pose, bending the knees with feet parallel, hips raised and chin to the sky. On exhale, lower the hips onto the mat, and gently roll into apanasana (see Benefits and Effects, page 23) to counterpose.

Intermediate Vinyasa, Sitting:
BENEFITS & EFFECTS

- In the sitting pose, dandasana (step 1) challenges the diaphragm to move towards the abdomen on inhalation, against the weight of the abdominal organs acting under the force of gravity.
- Inhalations with the arms rotated upwards and outwards open the chest and lung meridian. This encourages the pranic current (see page 12) and cultivates confidence and self-esteem.
- Deep exhalations help expel stale air, enhancing the eliminative/detoxification function of the body (apana vayu).
- The forward flexion of the forward bend encourages the breath into the back of the lungs.
- The belly push (step 4), purvottanasana, encourages the breath into the body. It stretches the front body and upper respiratory tract, focusing the breath into the upper thorax.

Intermediate Vinyasa, Standing

This sequence involves four pathways of movement: forwards (flexion), gentle backwards (extension), lateral (to open alternate lungs) and twists (to cleanse). If you experience dizziness or headache, rest longer in forward bend or move very slowly between stages, particularly when returning from the deep forward bend.

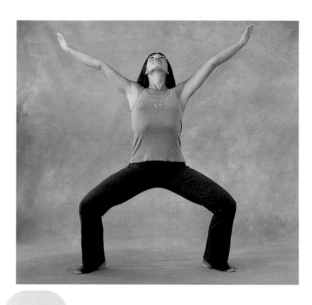

1 Stand in a wide stance with the toes slightly turned outwards and the legs straight. Inhale and stretch the arms high, bending your knees and turning them outwards. Simultaneously arc the arms forwards and diagonally out to the sides, while spiralling the arms outwards. Place particular emphasis on the thumb moving away from you.

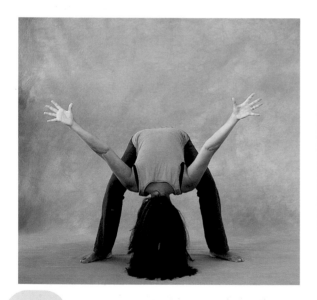

2 Now bend forwards from the hips and knees while exhaling deeply and spiralling the arms in the opposite way so that the palms face outwards with thumbs pointing to the sky.

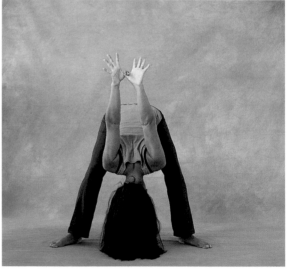

Additionally, hook the hands at the thumbs. Draw in the lower abdomen (uddiyana bandha) to reinforce the exhalation. Repeat both stages five to ten times, synchronized with the breath.

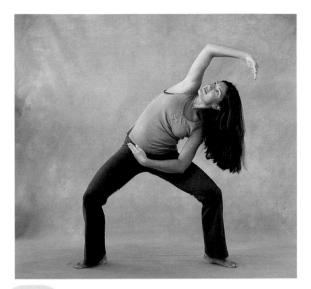

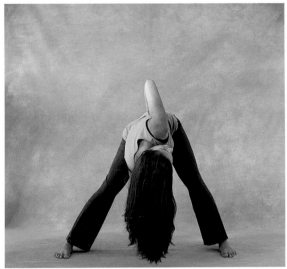

3 Return to the horse pose, with the arms outstretched to the sides. On exhale, arch the right arm overhead, lean to the left and arch the left arm under the belly to create a circular shape. Draw the right shoulder over the left shoulder for five breaths. Inhale and return to centre. Repeat on the other side to practise two full cycles on each side.

4 Stand with the legs straight and wide, and the feet parallel, arms outstretched to the sides. On inhale, lift and expand the chest. On exhale, pivot from the hips, placing the left hand on the floor in front of you and the right hand on the lower back, the sacrum. Use the right hand to monitor and limit any sacral tilting (imagine you can balance a teacup on the sacrum). Inhale, exhale and repeat on the other side.

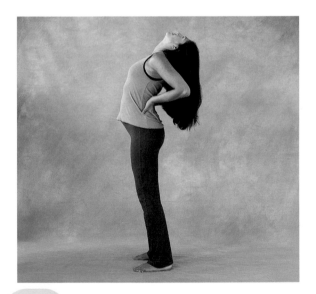

5 Stand with the feet hip-width apart and place the palms of the hands behind the pelvis with elbows pointing backwards. Inhale, lift the chest and take the chin upwards and backwards, allowing your back to arch slightly. Draw in the lower abdominal wall and place the tongue on the roof of the mouth to protect the neck. Exhale and return to centre. Repeat for five breaths but stop if you feel lightheaded.

 Intermediate Vinyasa, Standing:
BENEFITS & EFFECTS

- Inhalations with the arms rotated upwards and outwards open the chest area and lung meridian. This movement encourages the pranic current (see page 12) and helps to cultivate confidence and self-esteem.

- Deep exhalations with forward bends help expel stale air, enhancing the eliminative/detoxification function of the body ('langhana', apana vayu).

- When the hips are turned out and the arms outstretched, the front body, especially the chest and belly area, is opened, facilitating lung expansion and freedom of hara ('gut feeling').

- The squatting in the horse pose brings the major muscle groups into action – the gluteals, quadriceps and back muscles – which necessitate a high oxygen uptake. Deep breathing is thus stimulated.

Advanced Vinyasa

This sequence expands the whole chest cavity and facilitates deep breathing. It is particularly effective for relief from asthma, emphysema and bronchitis. The back bends combined with arm raises increase energy levels and boost self-esteem through encouraging deep inbreaths (prana current). If arm raises are too intense, practise this vinyasa keeping both hands on the ankles in step 4.

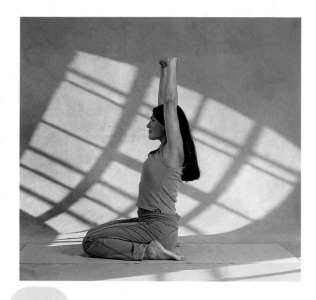

1 Sit in the thunderbolt pose, vajrasana, by lowering your buttocks between the inside surface of your feet with the heels touching the sides of the hips. Or simply kneel, or place a block under the hips for vulnerable knees. Lift the sternum to straighten the back and rest your hands on your knees, palms down. Inhale, raise arms above your head, palms to the sky and fingers interlocked, and breathe for ten breaths.

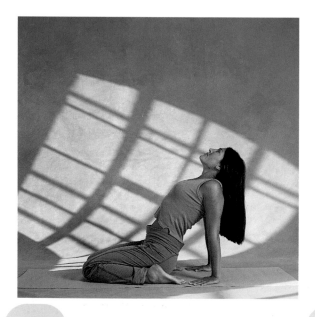

2 Now lean back with your palms flat on the floor behind you and the fingers facing forwards. Lift your chin towards the sky and breathe for eight deep breaths. Open the front wings of your chest. If necessary, elevate your hips on a block to protect your knees.

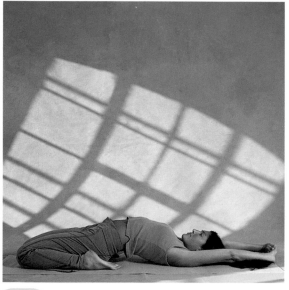

3 Gently lie back in reclining thunderbolt, supta vajrasana, as far as possible without strain. Try to keep your knees on the floor and pressed together. Tuck your tailbone under and deepen your inbreaths for 30 breaths. (You may like to end the practice here, in which case counterpose is child's pose, page 41.)

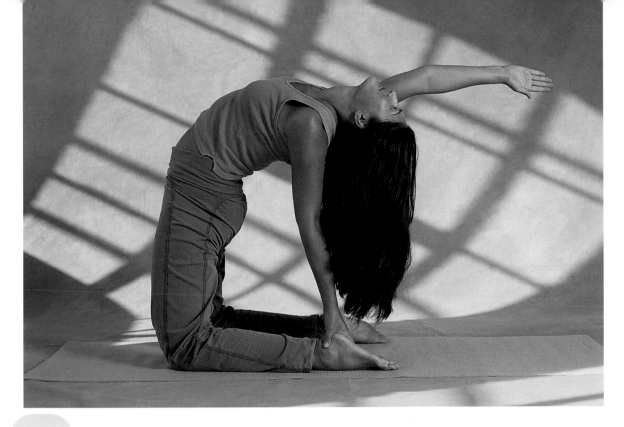

4 Return to the position in step 2, and lift your hips to prepare the camel pose (see page 41). Keeping the hips forwards, take a deep inbreath and lift the chest. Exhale, arch the back, catching your left ankle with your left hand and lifting your right hand to the sky. Do not crook your neck. Take eight breaths. If possible, arc the arm over the head to open the right side of the body. Inhale, return to raised kneeling: exhale, fold to child pose (page 41) or downward dog pose (page 40). Repeat on the other side.

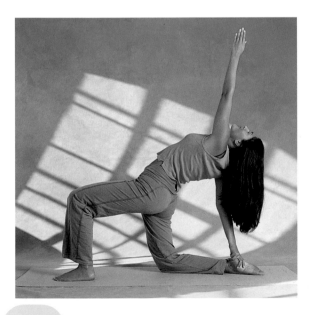

5 Now lunge the left foot forwards into the Warrior lunge. Exhale, plant the foot to earth. Inhale. Reach the left arm vertical to the sky as you lift up, placing the right hand on the right heel. Breathe for eight breaths. Repeat on the other side. Release to the child or downward dog pose.

Advanced Vinaysa:
BENEFITS & EFFECTS

- Raising one arm focuses the breath into alternate lungs by stretching the intercostal muscles – the muscles that lie between the ribs – and the sides of the waist on one side.
- The trachea (windpipe) is stretched and the respiratory muscles are challenged to siphon the air into the bronchii, which can help to dislodge mucus.
- The sequence introduces a full thoracic inhalation and perfusion of the alveoli as intrathoracic pressure peaks.
- Through the chest expansion exercises, the lungs are elevated.
- This vinyasa opens up the front body, abdomen and gut, removing stagnation.

Kapalbhati Breathing

This practice, meaning 'shining skull', is a breathing practice (pranayama) and a purification process (kriya), cleansing and reoxygenating the brain's frontal region. Avoid if you suffer from heart disease, high blood pressure, hernia or gastric ulcer.

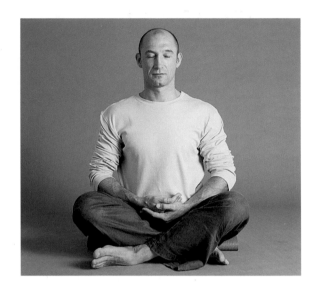

1 Seated in a comfortable pose with a straight spine, rest the hands on the knees or cup them in your lap (as shown right). Close the eyes and relax the whole body, drawing your intention to your breathing.

2 Inhale through both nostrils, expanding the abdomen. Then force the breath out through the nostrils while contracting the abdominal muscles towards the spine (like a concertina). Allow the inbreath to spontaneously fill the lungs and expand the abdomen without strain.

3 Repeat a strong, conscious exhale, contracting the abdomen inwards. Continue for ten breaths, then inhale and exhale deeply. This makes up one round. Practise three to five rounds.

4 On completion, meditate on the eyebrow centre (see page 122) and the frontal region of the brain.

Calming Belly Breathing

'Hara' breathing, or breathing into the gravitational centre of the body, is ideal to ease anxiety and stress. It is suitable for nervous, anxious people, particularly heart patients and asthmatics who tend to shallow breathe into the upper chest only. Belly breathing develops apana vayu, the eliminative pattern in the body (see page 12), and hence is detoxifying and relaxing. When Swami Rama

(1925–1996) visited the West he taught belly breathing and avoided the more stimulating thoracic breathing because he observed that Westerners needed to destress and centre themselves.

1 First, lie down in the corpse pose, savasana (page 23), with your arms by your sides. Inhale into the lower belly, feeling the navel rise and the sides of the waist and lower back expand. Fill only the lower lobes of the lungs.

2 Now exhale, emptying the lungs without force and observing the navel fall. Practise breathing for ten minutes. Meditate on the navel rising and falling.

Seated Spinal Twist

Twists 'wring out' the spine, relieving backache and massaging the abdominal cavity, in addition to expanding the lungs. This seated spinal twist – ardha matsyendrasana ('lord of the fishes') – nourishes the torso, including the chest cavity.

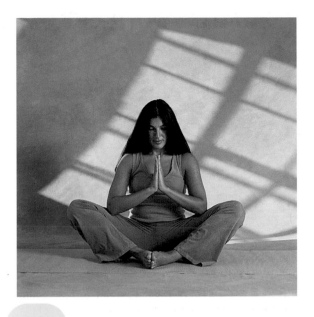

1 Sit with the soles of your feet touching and your hands in the prayer position, namaste. Rest your elbows on the upper thighs and breathe deeply for ten breaths.

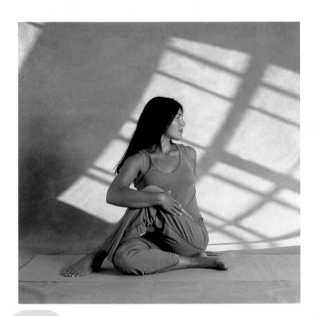

2 Now lift the left leg over the right knee, placing the left foot flat on the floor to the outside of your right thigh with your bent knee pointing straight up and your toes pointing forwards. Placing your right hand on your left knee and gently twist your torso to the left, lifting your chest to lengthen. Turn your head to the left and look over the left shoulder. Breathe freely and deeply, twisting and stretching the spine without strain for 8–20 breaths, focusing your breath into the left lung.

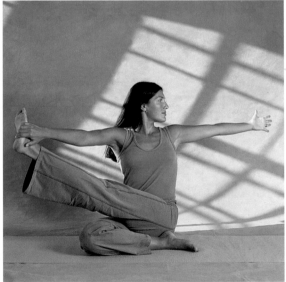

3 Now grasp your left foot with your right hand and stretch your leg outwards to straighten it, stretching your left arm in the opposite direction for a full open chest stretch. Hold for eight deep breaths. Repeat on the other side of the body. (Roll on your back in apanasana or curl to cosmic egg between sides, to return to symmetry (see pages 22 and 80.) Anchor your shoulderblades down your back to ease the shoulders away from the ears.

Prana Mudra

Learn to practise the whole sequence in one smooth inhalation, charting the flow of the breath through each stage. At the peak of the inhalation, retain the breath (khumbaka) and meditate on the energy coming in; on the exhalation, chart the flow of the breath to its source at the navel through the arm movements, reconnecting to your root.

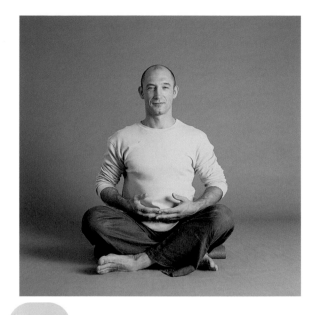

1 Seated in a quiet place with a straight spine, internalize your awareness by drawing attention to your breathing and spine. With broad shoulders, relax the face and lower the gaze to the nosetip or close the eyes. Cup your hands in your lower belly, palms upwards, and take a deep breath in, lifting the chest without straining. Breathe out, following your attention to mula bandha (root lock – see page 16). Contract the abdominal muscles gently as you empty the lungs.

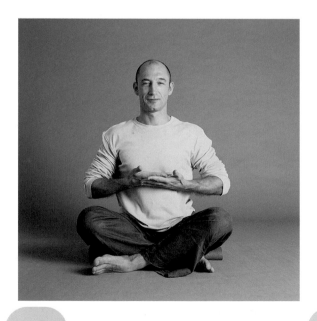

2 The abdominal phase: On the inhale, relax the belly and lift the hands up to solar plexus, charting the flow of the breath as it reaches and fills the lower lobes of the lungs.

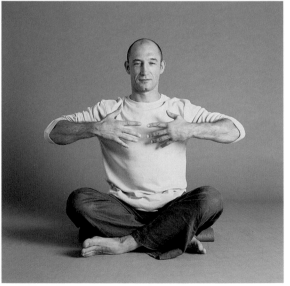

3 The thoracic phase: Continue to inhale, lifting the hands up towards the clavicles as you orchestrate the flow of the inbreath.

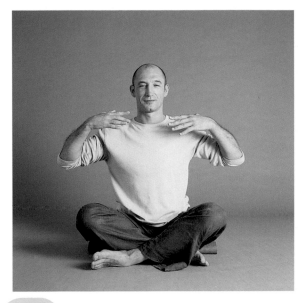

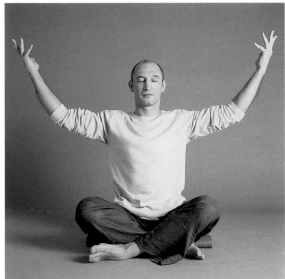

4 **The clavicular phase:** When you have nearly taken in a full inhale, spread the elbows wide in line with your shoulders, fingertips in front of your throat, to facilitate expansion of the chest (prana vayu). Pass your hands in front of your face, relaxing the face, internalizing your gaze with a serene expression.

5 At the peak of the breath, in an open gesture, open the arms and hands skywards. Retain the inbreath and visualize healing energy entering through the crown of your head, pouring down your spine and permeating every cell in your body. Beginning to exhale, slowly return the hands back to the start placing in your lap as you drain the lungs, and repeat.

Breathing:
BENEFITS & EFFECTS

- Prana mudra is a meditation on the complete, unrestricted breath, where expansive inbreaths are balanced with deep outbreaths.
- The hand gestures chart the journey of the breath, taking prana (energy) into any closed areas in the body and allowing greater awareness of breathing.
- Belly breathing slows down the heart rate and facilitates parasympathetic nervous system response, lessening hyperventilation, panic and asthma attacks.

Pranayama Practices

After your asana practice, it is a good idea to introduce ten to fifteen minutes of gentle breathing after a ten-minute relaxation period (savanasana). Practise the belly breathing and kapalbhati methods (see page 30) and practise ujjayi breathing (see page 120). For asthma, anxiety and hyperventilation, practise nadi shodana and bee breath methods (see pages 120–1).

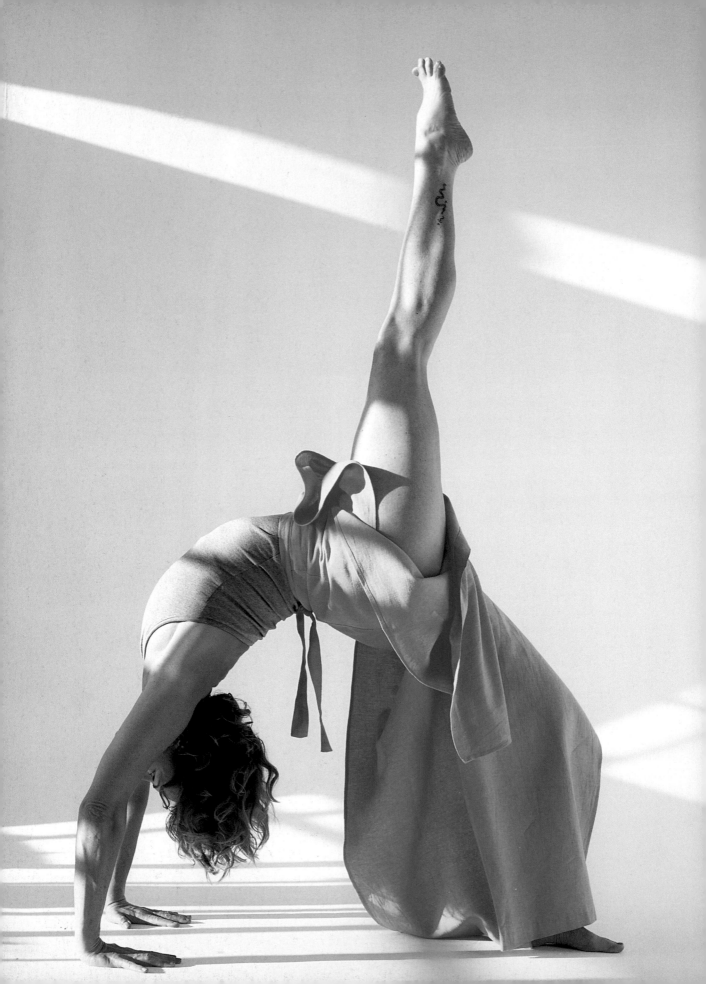

the neuro-endocrine complex:
the body's transmitters

The nervous system consists of complex networks of neurons (nerve cells) that carry information from the sensory receptors in glands, sense organs, muscles, and so on, to the central nervous system. Here they are processed, integrated and stored. Motor impulses are then transmitted to the appropriate organs in the body to effect action. The nervous system integrates and acts upon information from all the major systems of the body to maintain a stable internal environment – a condition known as homeostasis – and works closely with the endocrine system to achieve this.

Inappropriate activation of sympathetic arousal (known as the 'fight or flight' response) must be the most significant root cause of contemporary disease, due to the widespread effects it exerts on our physiology. In primitive life, sympathetic arousal was triggered by a threat to survival and was usually immediate and short-lived. Today, the response is usually concerned with work pressures or anxiety over financial or emotional issues, triggers we have come to refer to as 'stress'. Because our concerns cannot usually be resolved with immediate action, they persist as triggers for an unnaturally long, albeit mild, activation of the 'flight or fight' response. Yoga, by inducing the para-sympathetic response, lowers stress levels and thus calms the system.

THE AUTONOMIC NERVOUS AND ENDOCRINE SYSTEMS

The autonomic nervous system sends impulses from the central nervous system (within the brain and spinal cord) to the smooth muscle of the gut, the internal organs, the bronchii and lungs, blood vessels, the heart, glands and skin. Divided into two branches, which operate in response to our emotional states and immediate environment, it is regulated by centres in the brain such as the hypothalamus and brain stem nuclei.

The parasympathetic branch is active during times of rest and recovery and its purpose is to conserve and restore energy by directing blood flow to the internal body. This is the healing branch of the nervous system and a primary aim of yoga therapy is to encourage this modality. Unless impulses from the sympathetic nervous system override it, the parasympathetic system is dominant so that the everyday functions of digestion and metabolism can be carried out. The sympathetic branch of the autonomic nervous system is often referred to as the 'fight or flight' response and is activated to varying degrees when extra energy output is required.

Functionally related to the nervous system, the endocrine system works with it to maintain homeostasis. It is covered here so that the body's integrated response to stress can be better understood. The nervous system uses electrical impulses along neurons; the endocrine system uses chemical messengers (hormones). Thus, the endocrine system tends to be slower acting but longer lasting.

THE PHENOMENON AND PHYSIOLOGY OF STRESS

If stress persists, the body's follow-up response is stimulated and involves the endocrine system and the adrenal gland, in particular. The adrenal cortex responds to persistent stress by secreting two types of hormone. Mineralocorticoids increase blood volume by retaining sodium in case of blood loss. This has the effect of increasing blood pressure and can create hypertension. Glucocorticoids decrease the ability of the gut to absorb nutrients, but they also stimulate the release of calcium from bones, probably in anticipation of sustained muscular contraction. Calcium is used in neuromuscular conduction and contraction. If sustained, this metabolic disturbance may lead to osteoporosis.

Glucocorticoids (mainly cortisol) break down muscle and stored fat for energy leading to a rise in blood lipids and glucose. A sustained increase in circulating fats such as triglycerides, which uses a form of cholesterol (VLDL) as a carrier, can lead to atherosclerosis (thickening of the arteries)and increase the risk of coronary artery disease.

Prolonged stress also activates the thyroid gland, which controls and influences both general and organic metabolism by increasing the strength and rate of the heartbeat (further increasing blood pressure) and increasing the breakdown of glycogen and fat stores, elevating blood glucose still further. Elevated blood glucose levels (hyperglycaemia) are potentially damaging to the brain so the pancreas releases the hormone insulin to bring the level back to normal. The cells responsible for this function can eventually become exhausted, with permanent diabetes the likely result.

The stimulus to adapt to or withstand changes ('stresses') is surely one of the major driving forces of evolution and our survival as a species is partly due to our ability to respond to the myriad nature of stress, such as with fighting an infection. Even in a contemporary context a certain amount of stress is a spur to activity, helping us to cope with various challenges on our life journey and should not therefore be seen in an entirely negative light.

COMMON NEUROENDOCRINE DISORDERS

Osteoporosis is a reduction in bone mass, which may begin around middle age and occurs particularly in women after the menopause when levels of oestrogen fall dramatically. Potential causes are menopause, smoking, alcohol consumption, body composition (stored fat is a high source of oestrogen, which retards bone loss), calcium deficiency, long-term steroid or thyroid medication, some diuretics, lack of weight-bearing exercise and stress.

The connection between prolonged stress and osteoporosis can be easily overlooked. The endocrine system's response to stress is increased activity of the thyroid gland and the adrenal cortex, resulting in elevated levels of the hormones thyroxine and cortisol. Prolonged elevated levels can lower blood oestrogen levels and result in osteoporosis.

Hyperthyroidism, an overactive thyroid gland, can develop when the body responds to prolonged emotionally charged states by attempting to maintain a metabolic rate comparable to the degree of nervous system activity. Symptoms include increased heart rate, flushed skin, heat intolerance and weight loss. Potential causes are stress, artificial stimulants and a high-sugar diet.

Hypothyroidism, or an underactive thyroid gland, often follows an overactive thyroid and is a sign of the gland wearing out. Symptoms include a puffy face, slow heart rate, low body temperature, weakness and weight gain. The causes are the same as in hyperthyroidism.

Diabetes mellitus is manifest in two strains. Type 1, juvenile onset diabetes, is characterized by a lack or marked reduction of insulin-producing cells, requiring injections of insulin into the bloodstream. Type 2, mature onset diabetes mellitus, makes up approximately 90 per cent of cases and tends to occur after the age of 40. The signs are an elevated blood glucose level and a loss of glucose in the urine. Due to impaired kidney function, water reabsorption is poor, resulting in increased thirst to compensate for fluid loss. Potential causes of both types include a high-sugar diet from simple and/or refined carbohydrate and prolonged stress or emotionally charged states resulting in elevated blood glucose levels.

Pre-menstrual syndrome (PMS) is characterized by one or many features, such as depression, irritability, abdominal bloating, breast swelling/tenderness, food cravings, skin eruptions and backache, beginning about one week prior to the period. Potential causes are a diet deficient in essential fatty acids, excessive or prolonged stress, hormonal imbalance and dysfunction of the lumbo-sacral spine.

Multiple sclerosis (MS) is a progressive disease involving the destruction of the myelin sheaths of the nerves in the central nervous system, which develop multiple areas of scarring known as scleroses, effectively 'short-circuiting' nerve conduction. Symptoms can include visual disturbances, muscular weakness and diminished coordination. Potential causes include a post-viral infection precipitating an auto-immune response, a state when the body attacks its own cells (see also the immune system, pages 107–9).

Depression is a term applied to a wide range of negative emotions, from feeling unhappy to feelings of helplessness and thoughts of suicide. It appears to be linked with a reduction of serotonin and endorphins, and is an example of how our emotions and physiology are inextricably linked. Potential causes may range from physical illness or hormonal changes to the side effects of pharmaceutical or recreational drugs or social issues.

Insomnia is usually linked with stress, worry or depression, but may also be a side effect of pharmaceutical drugs such as beta blockers (for hypertension) or thyroxine (for hypothyroidism). Other causes include consumption of caffeine, alcohol and tobacco.

Headaches take many forms but the two most common are tension headaches and migraines. A persistent or recurrent headache that does not improve should be investigated medically. Tension headaches are usually due to local muscular tension in the neck, head, face and jaw. They can also be created by referred pain patterns. Migraines are usually of vascular origin and typically precipitated by 'triggers' such as caffeine, cheese, red wine and bright lights. Stress is an often overlooked trigger. Mechanical causes may also be involved. A common and often neglected cause of both types of headache is dehydration, a state that can take 48 hours to remedy due to the limits of kidney function.

THERAPIES AND TREATMENTS

Treatments include hormone replacement therapy (HRT) for osteoporosis, thyroxine for hypothyroidism, radioactive iodine or surgery for hyperthyroidism, analgesics/anti-inflammatory drugs for tension headaches, vasoconstrictors for migraines, immuno-suppressive therapy (glucocorticoids) for MS, dietary/exercise management in diabetes (or insulin in severe cases), analgesics/anti-depressants/ hormone therapy (usually as a contraceptive pill) for menstrual disorders and antidepressants for depression.

Lifestyle recommendations that may help include stress-reducing strategies. Eating sugary foods can invoke the stress response, so avoid foods containing a high proportion of sugars, which increase adrenaline production by up to four times. This applies to simple sugars and refined carbohydrates like white flour products and any food or drink containing caffeine. Perhaps most surprisingly of all, high blood glucose levels from excessive simple sugars increase the production of saturated fatty acids containing triglycerides. Buyers of low-fat foods should check the labels for sugar content as well as carcinogenic 'sweeteners'. Avoid smoking, which can also stimulate the stress response.

Although largely influenced by hormonal factors, yoga therapy for gynaecological disorders is covered in the genitourinary section (see pages 84–93). In addition to the following yoga practices, concentrate on the rehabilitation series (see pages 56–59) and chakra work (see pages 38–47). Also pranayamas will help the neuroendocrine system, especially bandha contraction on kumbhaka and the retention of outbreath (see nadi shodhana and ujjayi breathing on pages 120–1).

CHAKRA BREATHING MEDITATION

Seated in a comfortable meditation posture, such as sukkhasana, siddhasana or the lotus, practise ujjayi pranayama, the psychic breath (see page 120). Bringing your attention to the base of your spine, visualize your spine as the stalk of a lotus. As you breathe to the top of the stem (moving towards the top of the spine), imagine a brilliant flower forming, and around the stem, beautiful leaves. See tiny drops of dew-like pearls on the leaves which, if you shake them, fragment into beads. Become aware of the chakras, their related colours and their symbols. Locate them in your own body, visualizing them clearly in a way that resonates for you. Concentrate on each, exploring the qualities of element, energy and emotional connotation for yourself.

The chakras:

MULADHARA: located at the perineum and cervix; visualize a dark red lotus flower with four petals, symbolizing the earth – grounding.

SWADHISTHANA: at the end of the spine; visualize a vermilion lotus with six petals, symbolizing the concept of yielding.

MANIPURA: located behind the navel; visualize a yellow lotus with ten petals, symbolizing connection.

ANAHATA: located behind the heart; visualize a green lotus with 12 petals, symbolizing vision.

VISHUDDHI: located behind the throat, visualize a blue lotus with 16 petals, symbolizing perception.

AJNA: located behind the eyebrow centre; visualize a smoky grey lotus with two grey petals, symbolizing intuition.

SAHASRARA: located at the crown of the head; visualize a bright violet lotus radiating 1,000 petals.

Chakra Asana Practice

The following practice focuses on strengthening the chakras in ascending order from root to crown to stimulate the spinal nerves and cleanse the subtle body. For a full explanation of the chakras, with relevant breathing exercise, see page 43. It is essential to begin from earth (base of spine) and rise, anchoring spirituality in the mud of life, just as a lotus sends deep roots into muddy swamps.

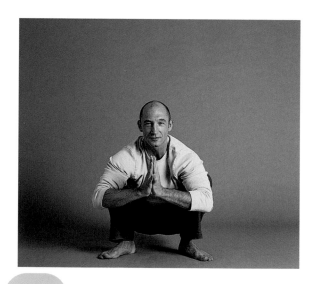

1 Place the feet hip-width apart and lower your body into a deep squat: your 'Indian armchair', the natural seat. Visualize the rooting energy of the earth and hold for ten breaths. Place the hands into namaste, the prayer position, and lift the chest.

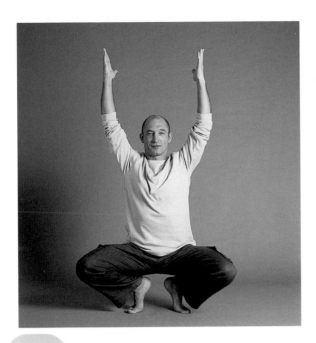

2 Inhale and lift the arms straight up, with palms facing each other. Open the hips and stretch the lower belly and groin. Balance on the balls of the feet. Visualize the ocean as you breathe into the pelvic region for ten breaths.

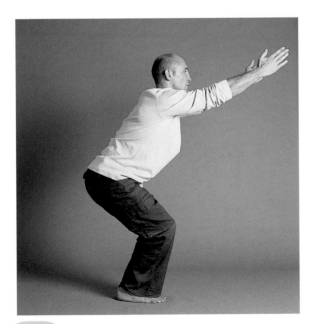

3 Inhale, bring legs together and rise to utkatasana, bending the knees. Squeeze the inner seams of the legs together, sweeping your arms forward. Keep the knees bent, drop the heels to the floor and anchor the tailbone.

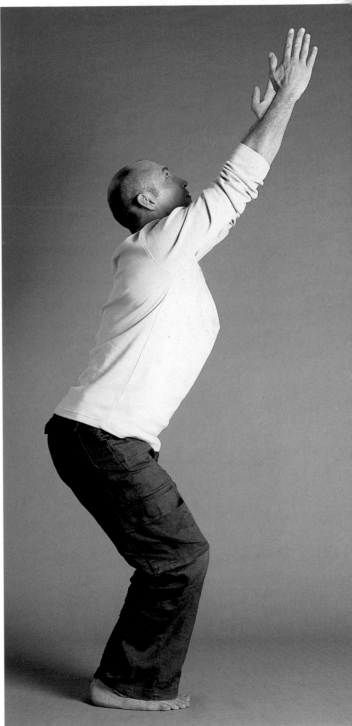

4 Ascend through the sides of the waist and trunk upwards to stretch the abdominal cavity. Visualize the sun, representing the digestive fire in the solar plexus, as you breathe for ten breaths.

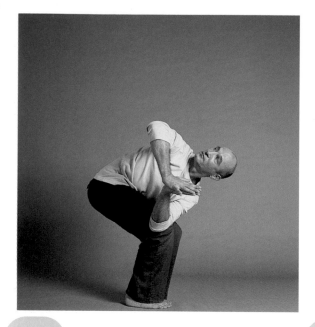

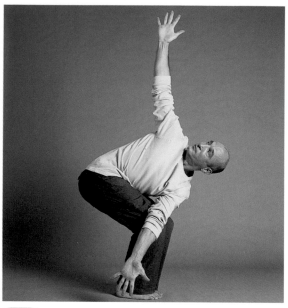

5 Now, on inhale, gather your hands to the heart. On exhale, twist to the right, anchoring the left upper arm outside the right thigh. Look up and draw your elbows away from each other. Pierce the sky with your right elbow. If you feel any tension in your neck, then look downwards.

6 On inhale, open arms vertically, expanding the chest and feeling the stretch upwards with your right arm and the downwards pull of your left. Visualize a massaging action of lungs around heart and take ten breaths. Repeat steps 4 and 5 on the other side. For a shorter sequence, end here in mountain pose, tadasana, breathing quietly (see page 52).

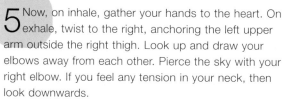

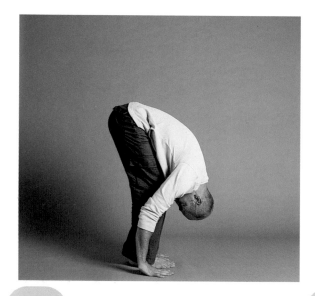

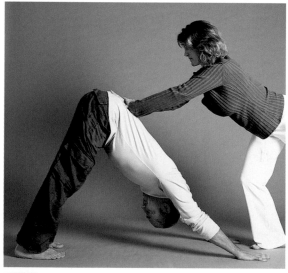

7 Exhale into a forward bend with feet and palms flat on the floor, lengthening the stretch through the hamstrings and lower back. Bend the knees in order to press and hollow the lower belly onto your thighs with each outbreath.

8 Move your hands forward and step into downward dog, adho mukha svanasana, rising on your toes, straightening your legs and lifting your hips to the sky. Make sure your head is released between your arms. Ground the heels without locking your knees.

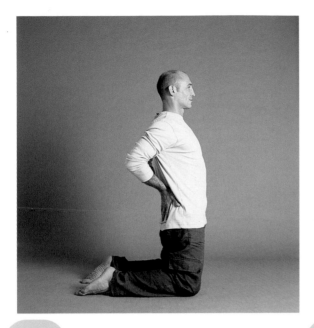

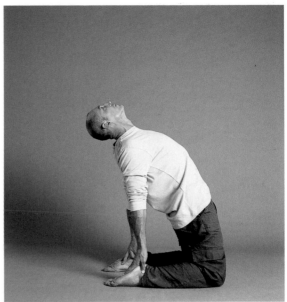

9 From downward dog, prepare for the camel pose. Kneel with your hips lifted and hands supporting your lower back with fingers pointed downwards and pressing downwards to create space around your lumbar. Draw your elbows back as far as you can, looking ahead. Inhale and lift the chest.

10 Inhale, lift the chest and keep the hips forward. Exhale, rest your hands on your ankles and arch the spine into the camel pose, ustrasana. Take your head upwards and backwards, keeping the mouth closed and the teeth slightly apart. Use your shoulders as a cushion to protect the neck. Visualize a rainbow arcing through the spine. Take ten breaths.

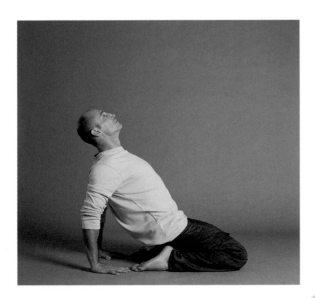

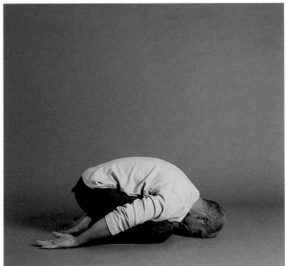

Modification: If you find the full camel in step 9 difficult, move into the hero pose, virasana, from step 8. Sit back on your heels and lean back, placing your hands behind you with elbows slightly bent.

11 Counterpose by folding forwards to rest in child's pose for ten deep breaths (see page 45). Feel the belly rise and fall against your thighs, let the shoulders drop like stones and take the breath into the back of the lungs.

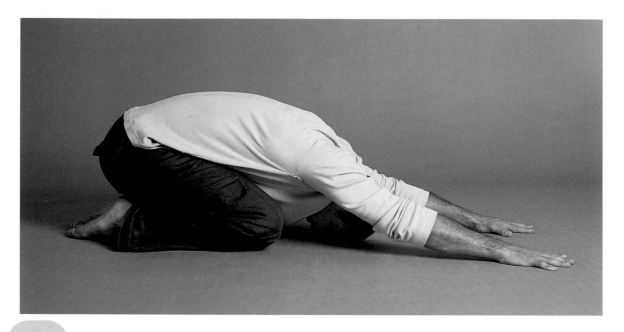

11 Extend your arms out in front of you to stretch the upper body. Breathe deeply into the side ribs to refresh the lungs, head and heart. For a shorter sequence, end here in child's pose (see page 45).

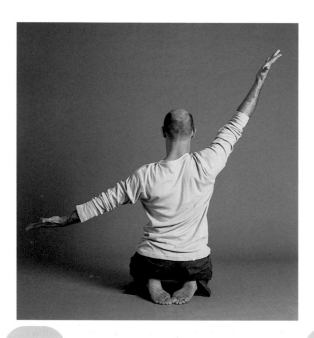

12 Now move into the sacred cow, gomukhasana. Sit in a kneeling position with the spine straight and your hands resting peacefully on your thighs. Raise your right arm to the sky and lower your left arm to the earth, feeling the diagonal pull through your limbs and opening out your chest.

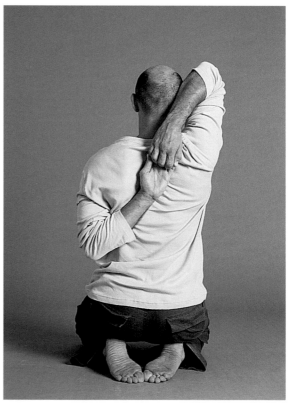

13 Bend your elbows and draw your hands behind your back to clasp the fingers together. Hold the position for five to ten breaths, then release. Lengthen the neck and gently anchor your tailbone under. Stabilize the pelvis and breathe with awareness.

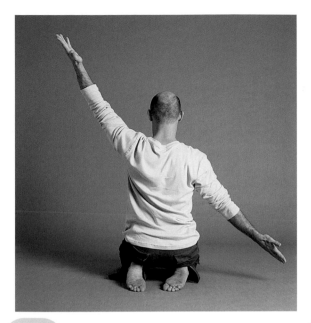

14 Raise your left arm to the sky and lower your right arm to the earth, repeating steps 12 and 13 on the opposite side of the body.

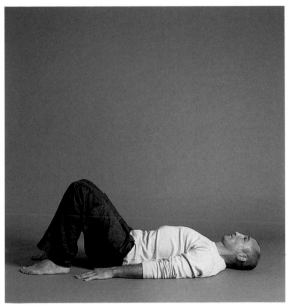

15 Now roll onto your back in preparation for sethubanda – pelvic lift. Lie on your back with your knees raised and arms by your side.

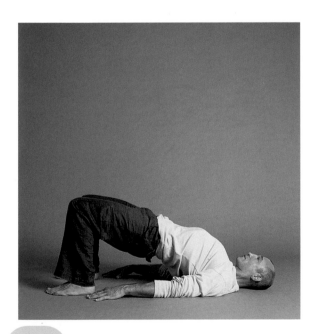

16 Inhaling, lift your lower body upwards in a pelvic lift, holding for ten breaths. Lower and repeat. This is a good preparation for the wheel, or peak pose (see page 44), or is a complete posture in itself. Counterpose in apanasana (see page 22).

Chakra Asana: BENEFITS & EFFECTS

- The squatting action in step 1 challenges the muscles of the pelvic floor, under the force of gravity, to maintain a cohesive resistance against the pelvic organs.
- The wide angle of the hips in step 2 creates space for prana to nourish the lower two chakras and the corresponding pelvic organs (see pages 14–15).
- Utkatasana in steps 3 and 4 opens up the solar plexus and stomach area, stimulating agni, the digestive fire, and the twisting action further massages this area.
- Backbends, including the camel and the wheel (see steps 9, 16 and overleaf), create space for the heart, corresponding to the anahata chakra.
- Inversions, as in steps 6 and 7, bathe the brain in oxygenated blood, nourishing the pineal and pituitary glands.

The Wheel

This can develop from step 16 of chakra asana (see page 43). Gomukhasana has prepared the shoulders to rotate, ready for this full extension, and backbends balance and tonify the neuroendocrine system.

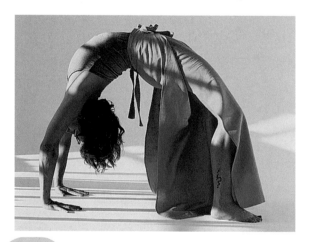

1 Lie semi-supine, with bent knees. Bend the elbows to the sky, placing the inner wrists beside the ears and the fingertips beneath the shoulders. Inhale, lift the chest and torso off the mat, straightening the arms. Keep the neck relaxed and feel the stretch throughout the entire front body. Hold for around ten breaths, spreading the work evenly throughout the spine.

Inversions
BENEFITS & EFFECTS

- Backbends, including the camel and the wheel, rejuvenate, energize and open the front of the body.
- They strengthen the arms, wrists, legs and ankles, and encourage life, vitality and ease in the spine.
- In addition to balancing the endocrine system, inversions help to decompress the lower spine and invigorate spinal circulation.
- This practice aims to integrate all the chakra energies progressively, starting from the root chakra and ascending through the spine.

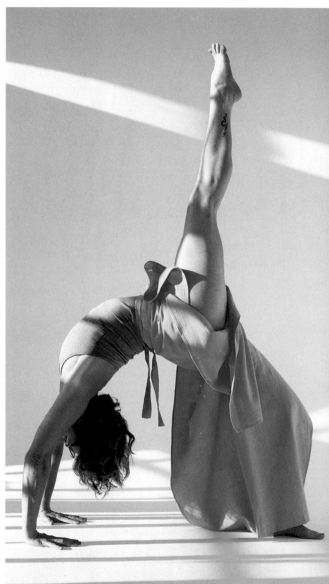

2 Now, if you can, lift your right leg towards the sky, keeping your left foot flat on the floor, knee directly above your ankle, and pointing your lifted toes. Visualize a rainbow arc through the smoothly arching spine, massaging the chakra wheels up to the throat. On exhale, release the right leg and change sides. Release the pose, relaxing into apanasana (see page 22) to counterpose. Deepen your outbreaths.

Child's Pose (Balasana)

This restorative pose can be used as a recuperative pause between the more challenging sequences. Balasana is also an essential counterpose for backbends. It helps relieve stress and fatigue, allowing you to reconnect inwardly, and it soothes lower back and neck pain.

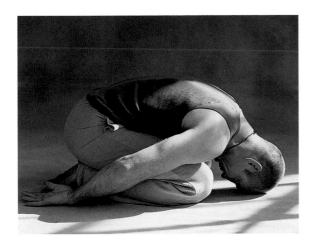

1 Kneel on the floor, sitting on your heels and touching your big toes together. On exhale, lower your upper body over your thighs, resting your forehead on the floor in front of you. Place your arms to your sides with the hands, palms up, near the feet. Relax your shoulders.

2 Allow the shoulder blades to separate and your spine to flex gently forwards. Rest in the pose until calm with steady, unencumbered breathing before lifting slowly back to kneeling.

Raised Child

For those who feel they do not have the strength or balance to support the full headstand position, try the raised child pose as a preparation. This is a safe approach to many of the same benefits as full inversions, bathing the upper body with oxygenated blood.

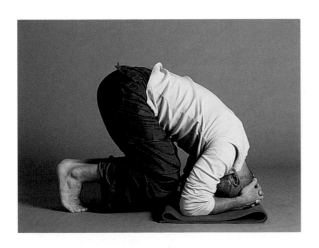

1 Prepare a padded based and kneel in front of it. Bend your elbows and cup the crown of your head with your hands, interlocking your fingers. Now place your head onto the padded base. (This is the preparation for the full headstand.)

2 On inhale, lift the torso up, balancing on the top of the head. Visualize the space around the neck as you breathe. Additionally, clasp hands behind your back and draw the arms up vertically.

3 Return to child's pose, bringing your arms back along your side. Observe the breath.

The 'King' Posture

This headstand posture, sirsasana, is an integrating, balancing inversion used to energize the neuroendocrine system and relates to the 'crown' chakra (see page 38). If you have difficulty practising the full headstand, remain in step 1, the raised child pose, until a teacher guides you into the pose.

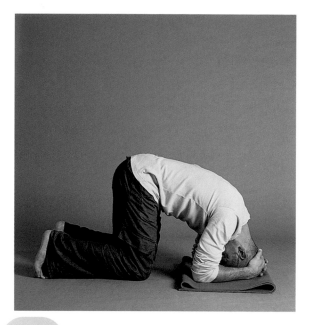

1 Prepare a padded base for your headstand. Kneel in front of the base, bend your elbows and cup the crown of your head with your hands, interlocking your fingers to create a forearm triangle. Place your head onto the padded base, hugging the back of the head.

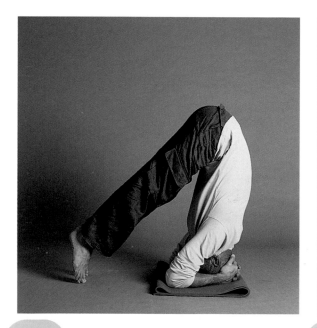

2 Keeping the neck long, lift the shoulders up from the ears. Straighten the legs. Tiptoe them into the body.

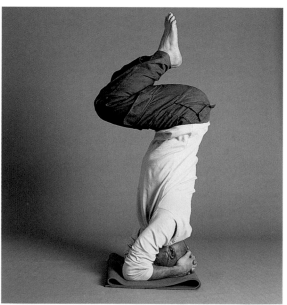

3 On inhale, and with the knees bent, lift the legs up, balancing the pelvis carefully above the shoulders.

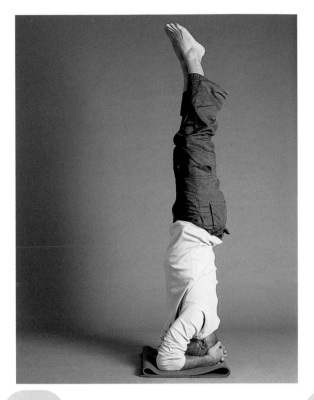

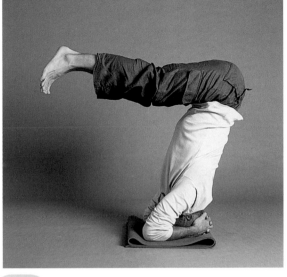

4 Inhaling, straighten your legs and hold for about 30 breaths. You may visualize a purple lotus flower at the crown of the head, with deep roots spreading throughout the body.

5 Now, if you can, lower your legs so they are parallel to the floor and hold for three to ten breaths. This cultivates uddiyana bandha, testing the 'gold' in your belly. Explore the pelvis as the fulcrum of your movement.

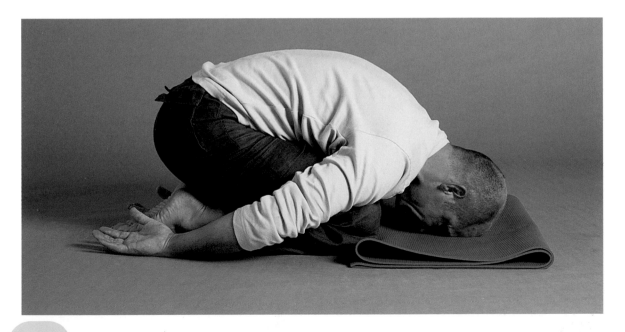

6 Exhale and lower your feet to the floor with control through the use of the bandhas, as in step 2 and counterpose in child's pose (see page 45) to rest and restore.

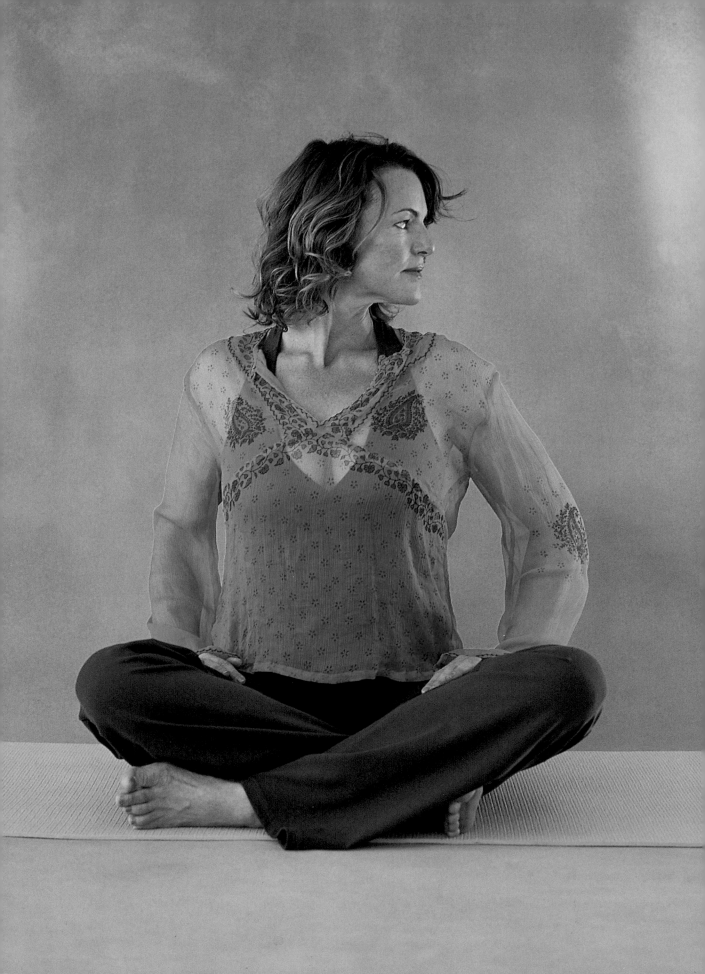

the cardio-vascular system:
the divine spark

The yogis located the seat of consciousness to reside in the cave at the back of the heart, which they named 'jyoli', the eternal flame or 'divine spark'. Yogis considered the heart to be the seat of the consciousness, not the head. In yoga practice we draw the mind into the heart by following the thread of the breath, floating the mind upon the breath as a lotus flower floats upon the water.

The cardiovascular system is the body's transport system, made up of the heart, the blood and countless blood vessels. The heart is a muscular, chambered pump, which powers the dynamics of blood circulation via the blood vessels. Together with the heart, the blood vessels, form a closed network of tubes that transport fluid to all parts of the body (arteries carrying oxygenated blood to the tissues and veins carrying deoxygenated blood back to the heart). As its primary role the blood transports oxygen and nutrients to the body's million of cells and removes waste products and carbon dioxide from them. Wherever blood is distributed. In a healthy body, it is able to carry out these functions.

THE HEART

A hollow, muscular organ, the heart beats over 100,000 times a day, pumping 7,000 litres (over 12,000 pints) of blood through almost 100,000 km (over 60,000 miles) of blood vessels. The heart is encased in a two-layered sac called the pericardium, which is cushioned between the lungs. The outer layer of the pericardium is anchored to the chest (sternum) at the front and the diaphragm beneath. It has a fluid-filled cavity that permits expansion of the heart with each contraction, while minimizing friction with the body wall. Cardiac muscle (myocardium) is considered involuntary in medical science. However, it has been proven that some experienced yogis can use it at will to control their heartbeat.

The heart has four chambers: two atria, which receive blood and two ventricles, which pump out blood. The right atrium receives deoxygenated, venous blood, which is then pumped, via the right ventricle, into the lungs for reoxygenation. The left atrium then receives the oxygenated blood from the lungs and pumps this, via the left ventricle, into the arteries for circulation. There are four valves in the heart that prevent backwards flow, both between the atria and ventricles, and at the ejection points of the ventricles themselves.

THE BLOOD AND ITS FUNCTIONS

Blood is composed of many dissolved substances and cells in a fluid known as plasma. Although 90 per cent water, plasma also contains proteins that play important roles in the immune system, blood clotting and osmotic pressure. Plasma also contains regulatory substances such as hormones and enzymes, food substances such as amino acids and some respiratory gases. Red blood cells contain iron pigment called haemoglobin, which is responsible for the blood's ability to carry oxygen. White blood cells combat inflammation and infection, and platelets are responsible for blood-clotting, a vital response to injuries that prevents excessive blood loss. Blood is the fundamental means through which the body's various organs and systems communicate with each other. Its functions are listed below.

- **Transport** The blood carries oxygen from the lungs to the cells and carbon dioxide away from the cells to the lungs. It transports nutrients from the gut to the cells and carries waste products away from the cells. Through it, hormones travel from the endocrine glands to the cells and metabolic heat is carried away from cells.
- **Regulation** The blood regulates body temperature through water content, and regulates water content

of the cells through sodium and potassium. It also stabilizes the pH level (acid/alkaline balance).
- **Protection** White blood cells and specialized proteins help the immune system and protect against infection. Platelets guard against blood loss through their clotting mechanism.

THE CIRCULATORY SYSTEMS

The sequence referred to as the systemic circulation carries oxygenated blood through large arteries from the heart's left ventricle, before dividing into medium- and smaller-sized, muscular-walled arteries and finally, into even smaller vessels known as arterioles. The arterioles then branch into microscopic vessels called capillaries. At the capillary bed/cell membrane interface, numerous substances are exchanged between the blood and the body's cells due to differences in both fluid pressure (hydrostatic pressure) and differences in concentration of solutes (osmotic pressure). Capillaries merge at this point to form small veins known as venules, which carry the now deoxygenated blood and cellular waste products. These venules in turn converge to form larger veins, notable for their important valves to prevent the backflow of blood. The venous system then terminates in the right atrium of the heart.

The two main subdivisions of the systemic circulation are the coronary circulation, which fuels the cardiac muscle, and the hepatic portal circulation, which directs venous blood from the gut (intestine), stomach, pancreas and spleen to the liver. The pulmonary circulation is the vital pathway via which venous blood is oxygenated in the air sacs of the lungs and returned to the heart.

BLOOD PRESSURE

Our blood pressure is influenced directly by the rate and force of our heartbeat and the consequent pressure exerted on the blood vessel walls. The size of the vessels' internal space (lumen) and the elasticity of their walls are also key factors. Clinically, blood pressure is measured in the arterial system, as it is higher here than in the veins and therefore more relevant as an indicator of health. Blood pressure is written as systolic blood pressure/diastolic blood pressure. The average for a young healthy adult is 120/80 mmHg (mercury).

Blood pressure can be altered immediately by certain chemicals, emotions and exercise and can also be changed over a longer term by a sustained unhealthy diet. To keep it within fairly narrow limits, nature has evolved ingenious devices within both the nervous and the circulatory systems.

If blood pressure becomes too low it can create light-headedness; if too high, there is risk of haemorrhage. Blood pressure is controlled by centres in the brain stem and by receptors in the carotid artery, aorta and right atrium of the heart. With reference to yoga asanas, the carotid sinus reflex and right atrial (heart) reflex are most relevant. In all inversions, when the heart is higher than the head, the carotid sinus reflex will reduce blood pressure and heart rate because arterial pressure in the neck is increased. This also works in reverse if arterial blood pressure in the neck falls, such as when you stand up after lying down. This reflex is activated in both ways during the sun salutation (see pages 52–55), which helps balance blood pressure. Full inversions are contra-indicated in cases of medium to high blood pressure or in rehabilitation following heart problems or strokes.

COMMON CARDIOVASCULAR DISORDERS

In addition to the conditions described below, more common conditions are disorders that vary in severity and are usually the underlying cause of the conditions listed. In their acute form, these conditions are medical emergencies and should be treated as such. However, in the rehabilitative phase of recovery, with medical consent, yoga therapy can be carefully introduced.

A stroke occurs from disorders of the blood vessels which supply the brain and results in the destruction of brain tissue. Usually affecting one side of the body, symptoms include the loss of limb function, slurred speech and coordination problems.

Myocardial infarction, commonly known as a heart attack, occurs when there is interrupted arterial blood supply to the heart, and cell death of the heart muscle occurs. Symptoms include severe chest pain, which may radiate down one or both arms.

Coronary artery disease is the condition in which the heart muscle receives inadequate blood supply from its arteries. It is characterized by chest pain, at rest or brought on by exertion. In angina, chest pain is usually accompanied by pain in the left arm or shoulder.

Arteriosclerosis is the process by which fatty substances are deposited in walls of arteries. It can lead to vascular spasms causing hypertension, stroke and coronary heart disease.

Hypertension, or high blood pressure, is most commonly caused by stress and a diet high in sodium. It increases the likelihood of heart attacks and strokes and can eventually damage the eyes and kidneys. Symptoms include an increased force in heartbeat and dizzy spells.

Hypotension, or low blood pressure is characterized by lightheadedness and can have inherited causes.

Deep vein thrombosis occurs when a blood clot appears in a vein, most often in the deep veins of a leg. Symptoms are throbbing pain and hotness, and causes can be hypertension, arteriosclerosis, trauma, long-haul flights and postsurgical bed rest.

Varicose veins are characterized by the swelling and/or distension of a vein due to pooling of venous blood. An inherited predisposition, long periods of standing, a lack of exercise and pregnancy are all possible causes.

THERAPIES AND TREATMENTS

Orthodox treatment for hypertension includes beta-blockers to slow down the heart rate and diuretics to reduce the plasma content and, therefore, volume of blood. In addition, both are used to reduce blood pressure, although side effects include disturbance of sleeping patterns and a reduction in the metabolic rate. Other conditions are treated with artificial vasodilators (agents that cause the walls of blood vessels to expand), anticoagulents (blood thinners) and anticholesterol drugs.

Lifestyle recommendations that may help are:
- Plenty of aerobic exercise, such as walking, jogging and swimming, at an appropriate intensity for your condition, carried out at least three times per week
- Avoid stimulants that can trigger the sympathetic nervous system, resulting in increased blood pressure. Caffeine, sugar and tobacco are all main culprits but also keep salt to a minimum in the diet
- Garlic and omega 3 essential fatty acids (EFAs) found in oily fish and seeds, can reduce blood fats, thereby lowering the risk of arteriosclerosis.

The role of yoga is to increase our psychological and physiological capacities to resist stress on the heart through psychophysical practices. Sattwic – balanced living habits – is linked with nature, thereby introducing contemplation and relaxation into life. Try to perform daily asanas from those listed in this chapter, for 20 minutes to an hour each morning and evening, followed by pranayamas (see pages 120–1) to restore the natural rhythm of the heartbeat. Yoga nidra (see page 123) provides a deep relaxation that soothes and stabilizes the heart, removing anxieties and stress triggers.

Sun Salutation
(Suryanamaskar)

The sun salutation can be practised by everyone as it may be adapted to individual needs, although it is not for those with moderate to high blood pressure. Traditionally practised at dawn as a bodily prayer before other postures, the sun salutation is accessible to all ages and consists of a standard series of movements.

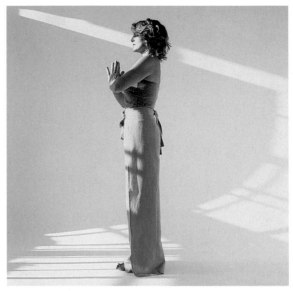

1 Stand in the mountain pose (tadasana) with the feet together and the spine straight. Take a deep, full breath. Exhale and place the hands in prayer position (namaste).

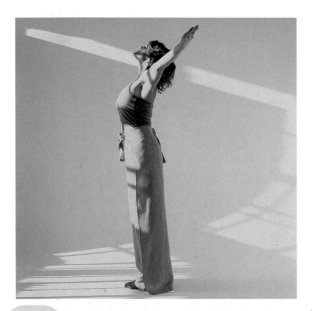

2 Inhale and reach the arms up over the head, lengthening the spine and looking upwards. Open out the arms, stretching through the chest.

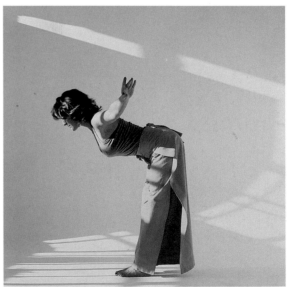

3 Exhale and fold halfway into a forward bend, keeping your spine parallel to the floor.

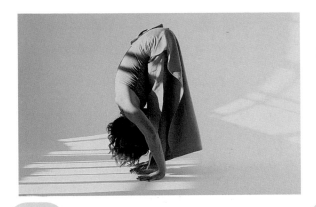

4 On full exhale, bend fully, placing the palms flat on the floor beside the feet. Bend the knees if the back or hamstrings feel tight.

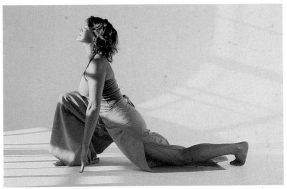

5 Inhale and lunge the left leg back, so that the left knee is placed on the floor. Look up and let your fingers touch the floor to either side of your right foot.

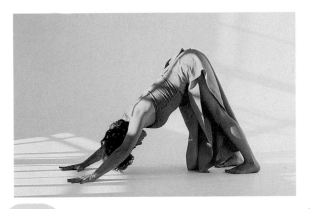

6 As you exhale, palms pressed to floor, bring the right leg back into the downward dog pose (see page 40), with the hips extending to the sky.

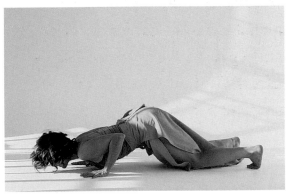

7 Exhaling, drop the knees to the floor and gently lower the chest to the floor between the hands. The chin or forehead rests on the floor.

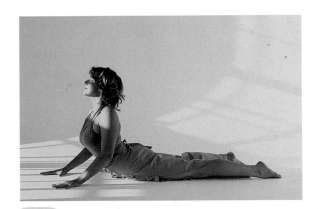

8 Inhale and slide the body forwards and upwards, arching the spine into cobra. With the stomach stretched and chest open, look up while the legs remain on the floor. (Your palms are flat on the floor in front of you, fingers spread like a starfish.)

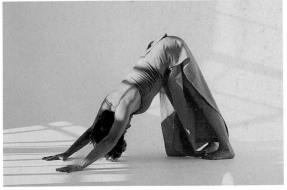

9 Exhale, press the hips back into downward dog, dropping the head between your arms and press the heels into the floor.

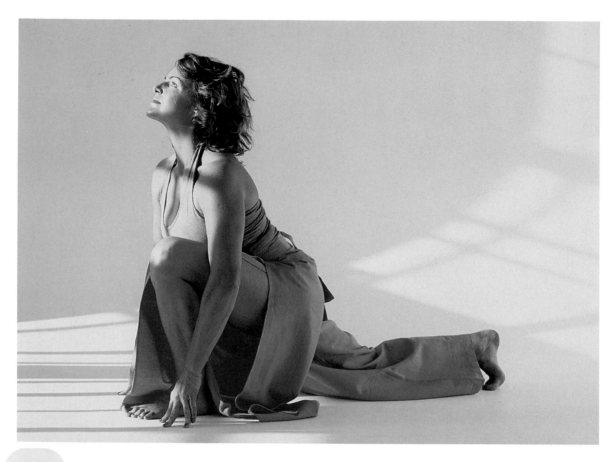

10 Inhale, place the left foot forwards between the hands, dropping the right knee to the floor. Look upwards.

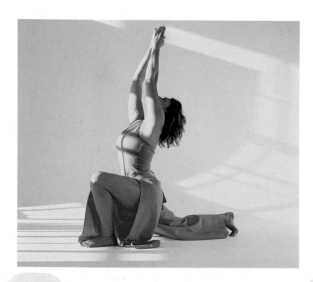

11 Sweep your arms up, letting your head rise with your arms, until, palms together, your hands are raised skywards.

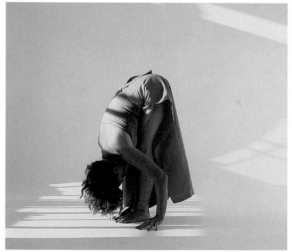

12 Exhale, step forwards with the right foot, placing it beside the left. Fold into a standing forward bend, head to knees.

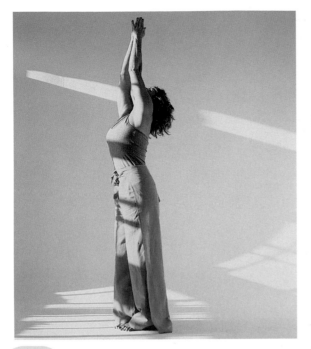

13 Inhale and sweep your upper body skywards, reaching the arms up over the head. Look up and lengthen the spine.

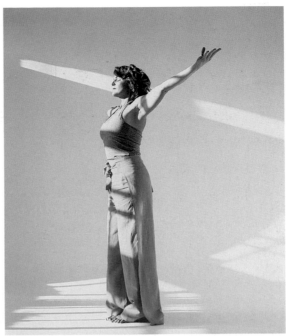

14 Sweep your arms out to the side and open out your chest.

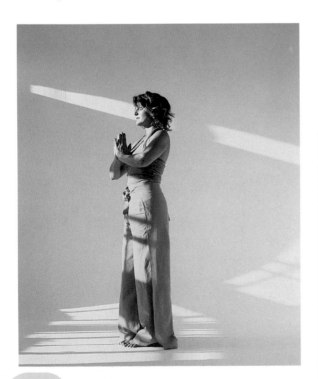

15 Exhale, release the arms and bring them back to prayer position – namaste.

Sun Salutation:
BENEFITS & EFFECTS

- The sun salutation activates the heart and increases circulation throughout the body.
- It is an excellent practice to normalize blood pressure and improves coordination and respiratory function.
- The alternating orientation of the head, heart and legs challenges the cardiovascular reflexes to adapt to the fluctuations in blood pressure, particularly in the head.
- Hypotension (low blood pressure) improves efficiency in maintaining optimal arterial pressure.
- Stretches all the major muscle groups in the body on all sides. Works up the entire body and rejuvenates.
- Sun Salutation is a prayer for the body to greet the sun as a symbol of 'buddhi' – untainted shining intellect/higher mind.
- Creates internal roots and stability – groundedness.

Rehabilitation Series

These slow, simple, rhythmic exercises orchestrated on the breath integrate psychophysical connections and can be used in rehabilitation in a hospital bed or in a seated position, although they are not recommended for acute cases. In addition to being suitable for the recovery phase from heart attack, stroke and surgery, they also help with infections and severe incapacities such as advanced emphysema.

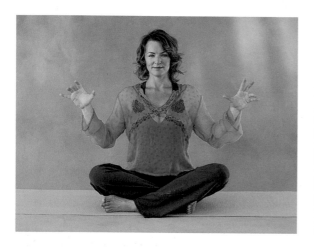

Finger Stretch: Move the fingers of both hands in spidery movements as if you are playing the piano for ten breaths.

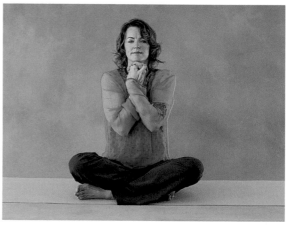

Wrist Stretch 1: Flex, extend and rotate each wrist. Then, clasping your hands together, cross your wrists left over right, and fold your arms under your chin.

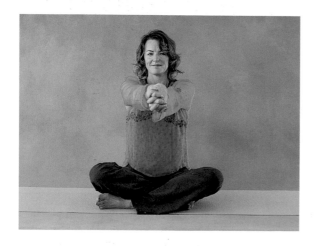

Wrist Stretch 2: Stretch your arms out in front of you, wrists still clasped, to limber the joints in the arms.

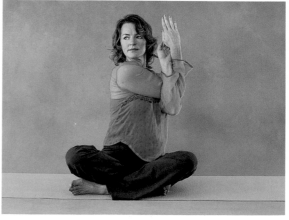

Wrist Stretch 3: Hook the right elbow over the left. Draw arms to the left and gaze to the right. Repeat to the right.

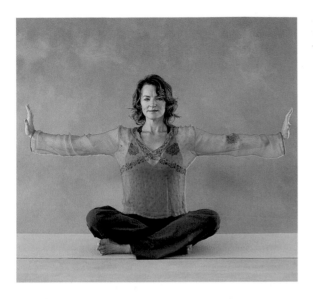

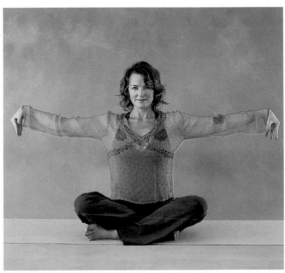

Wrist Flexion: With the palms facing the floor, extend your arms out to the sides. On inhale, flex the hands so the palms are facing away from the body; on exhale, point the fingers down. Continue for five breaths.

Wrist Rotations: Keeping your arms out to the sides, rotate your wrists by circling the hands, from the wrists, in both directions for five full rotations (you can do this without arms outstretched).

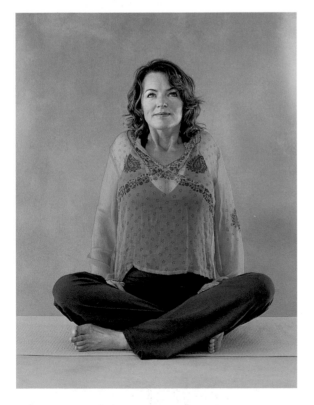

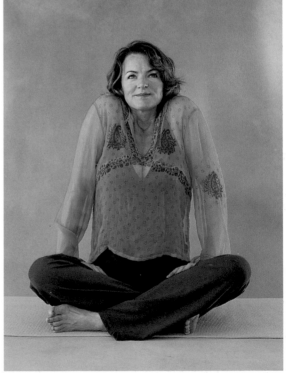

Shoulder Release: Look straight ahead, relax your neck and press your palms firmly onto your inner thighs. On inhale, rotate your shoulders up to the ears, then on exhale draw them slowly down, sliding your shoulder blades down your back. Repeat five times in each direction. Aim to straighten your arms as you lift your shoulders up towards the ears, thus pressing your thighs.

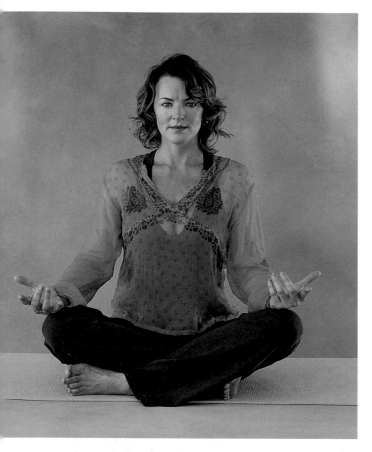

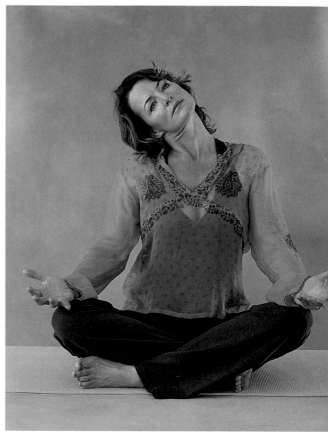

Neck Release: Look straight ahead and relax your neck (see above). On exhale, drop your right ear to your shoulder, come to centre and then drop your left ear to your shoulder (see above right). Repeat three times. On exhale, look to your left, inhale, return to centre and look to your right (see below right). Repeat three times.

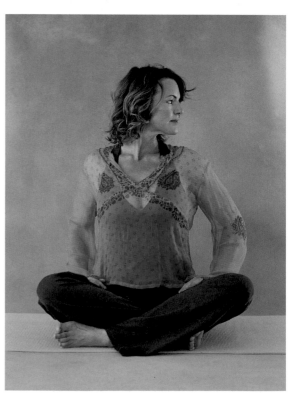

✳ Rehabilitation:
BENEFITS & EFFECTS

- Addresses all conditions, especially for circulation and nerves.
- Activates the brain, stimulates the peripheral circulation and removes sluggishness.
- Hand, foot and face movements stimulate the majority of the brain's motor cortex.
- Eye exercises stimulate the brain's integrative pathways and induce concentration.
- The eyebrow gaze (shambhavi mudra) balances the right and left hemispheres of the brain.
- The tongue extension in the Lion stretch cleanses and refreshes the pharynx and tongue.
- Shoulder movements shed accumulated tension.

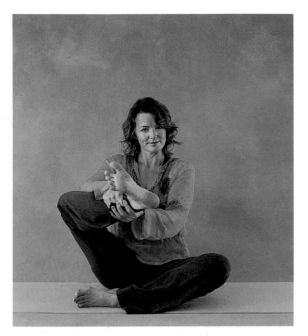

Foot Stretch: Bend and flare the toes of each foot five times. Flex and extend your feet five times, then rotate the ankles in a circle in both directions. Repeat five times on the other foot.

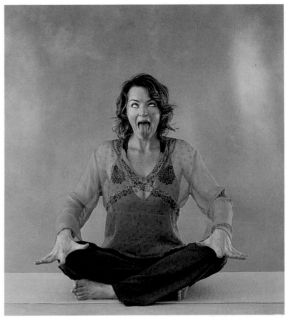

Lion stretch: Inhale deeply. Exhale, stick out the tongue, stretch the face and look up. Stretch your fingers like lion's claws. Hold momentarily and contract mula and uddiyana bandha (see pages 16–17).

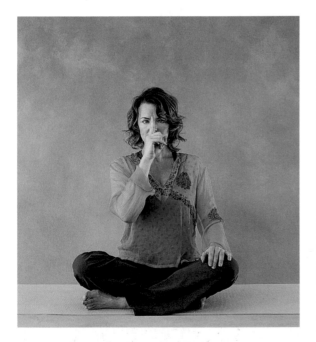

Eye Exercises: Keeping the head steady, look up, down and to both sides. Repeat three times. Place a finger in front of your nose at arm's length, with your other hand resting on your thigh, and watch the finger as you draw it towards the bridge of your nose and

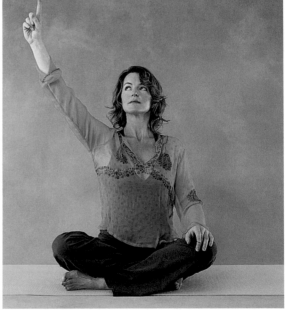

then away again. Repeat five times. Now, with both hands on your left knee, follow the finger of your right hand as you move it diagonally across your body to the uppermost right point you can reach with your right hand. Repeat on the other side with the other hand.

Basic Supine Vinyasa

This is a beginner's sequence that is especially suitable for cardiac and stroke rehabilitation. Practise each movement mindfully, step by step, connecting breath with movement. Do not force any movement.

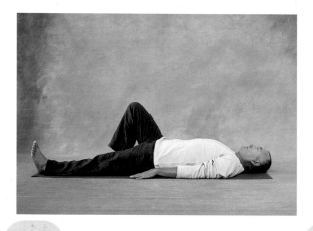

1 Assume the corpse pose (savasana, see page 122). Lie flat on the floor and place your arms alongside the body with shoulders relaxed away from the ears. Observe your breath. On exhale, bend the right knee until the sole of the foot rests on the floor.

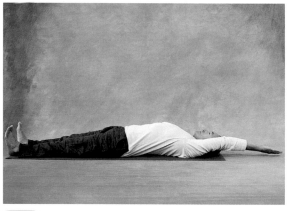

2 On inhale, straighten the right leg and bring the left arm up over the head. Repeat five times with the right leg and left arm alternating.

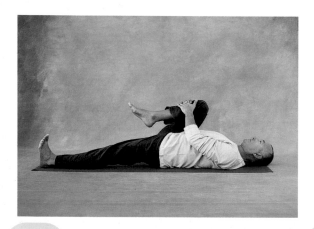

3 Exhale, bend the right knee and, with the left arm, squeeze the thigh to the abdomen, breathing out fully. Now repeat with the left leg and right arm.

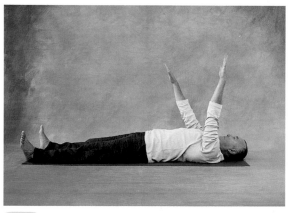

4 Inhale, raise your right arm over your head, without straining, and then on exhale, release. Repeat with the left arm. Then alternate arms, one raising and one lowering, simultaneously. Inhale and lift both arms up over the head. On exhale release the arms back to the sides. Repeat five times.

Intermediate Supine Vinyasa

A slight variation on the basic supine vinyasa, this is also suitable for rehabilitation of heart and stroke problems as it gently improves the blood circulation in the body.

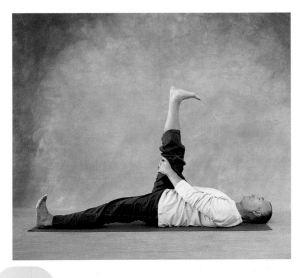

1 Repeat steps 1 to 3 of the Basic Supine Vinyasa, page 60. On inhale, place your hands around the back of the right thigh for support, attempting to straighten your right leg to the sky.

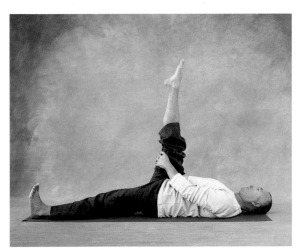

2 Flex and point your right foot five times on inhale.

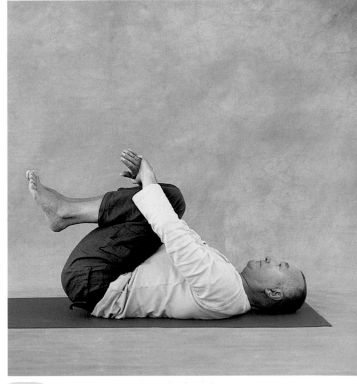

3 Exhale, bend your knees and squeeze your thighs to the abdomen. Switch legs and repeat with your left leg. Continue for up to five times for each leg. Stop if your breathing cycle becomes erratic. Return to the corpse pose, savanasana (see page 122).

Advanced Supine Vinyasa

Suitable for mild hypertension and angina. However, avoid this sequence if you suffer from moderate to high hypertension or you are recovering from recent cardiac problems or a stroke. If you experience increased pressure or discomfort in the head, elevate your head on a pillow. If chest pain or breathing difficulties arise, stop immediately.

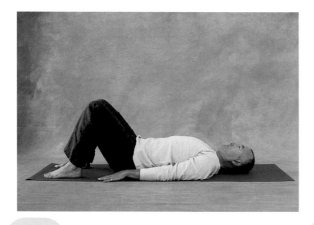

1 Rest in the corpse pose, savasana (see page 122) and observe your breathing. Assume the semi-supine position, knees bent and feet hip-width apart with arms, palms down, by the sides. Take a relaxed abdominal inbreath.

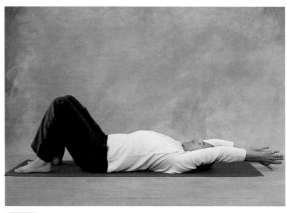

2 On inhale, raise your arms up over your head.

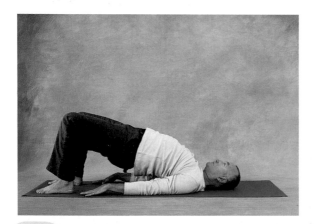

3 Exhale. Bring your hands down to your sides and simultaneously lift the pelvis. On inhale, lower the hips back down while raising your arms up over your head. Repeat up to five times. Rest in semi-supine.

Supine Vinyasa: BENEFITS & EFFECTS

- Leg squeezes increase abdominal pressure, enhancing venous return from the abdominal blood reservoirs.
- Vertical leg raises further increase venous return without overloading the heart.
- Alternately pointing and flexing the ankle activate the pumping action of the calf muscles to squeeze venous blood towards the body. This is very beneficial for varicose veins.
- The action of the diaphragm in step 3, left, pumps the livers and spleen, which are both important in managing the constituents of the blood.

Coronary Rest
(Supported Savasana)

Savasana means corpse, a condition of dropping resistance, inducing dynamic stillness and thus self-healing and self-acceptance. The nerves are eased, anxiety is reduced, blood pressure is lowered and depression is lifted. This supported version rests the heart, improves cardiac performance and can be practised in bed, with the head and legs elevated by pillows, to facilitate venous blood return to the heart from the legs, avoiding headache or dizziness. It is also ideal for pregnancy. Relax in this state of surrender and ease for a minimum of ten minutes after your asana practice.

Visualization:

This heart-healing visualization is directed at channelling healing energies (prana, positive thought power and bioenergy) to renew and replenish the blood vessels. Begin by concentrating on the navel centre, and direct your breathing there. Imagine golden light pooling and spreading from the Manipura chakra, the navel centre (see page 38) and, as you inhale, move awareness from navel to heart, like a comet trailing golden light. Pool this warm energy inside the heart, and imagine this light beginning to suffuse the blood vessels, to spread through the body in veins of gold, seeping into the muscles and cells as if you are enshrined in a golden cocoon. Feel the blood being charged and purified with each breath, infusing the whole body ... and the whole body cleansed.

Lie flat on the floor with the head and feet elevated slightly on pillows. Allow the feet to fall outwards, slightly apart. Close the eyes, allowing them to descend towards the back of the skull and dropping awareness from the conscious (front body) to the unconscious (back body). Now follow yoga nidra (see page 123), using the heart-healing visualization exercise described above.

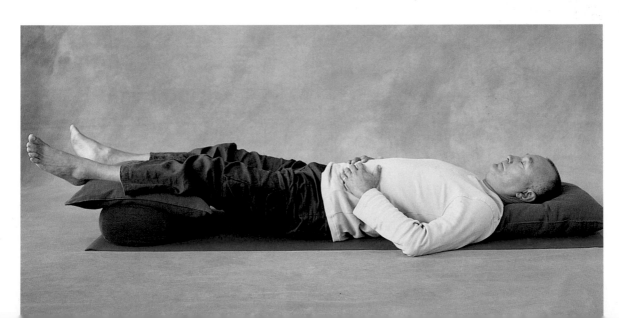

Advanced Plough Raises

Combining the plough, halasana, with alternate leg raises drains venous blood from one leg at a time, thereby improving blood flow back to the heart without overloading it.

For an easier modification, keep your knees bent throughout the exercise and support your lower back with your hands. Do not strain but lift your legs slowly and gently.

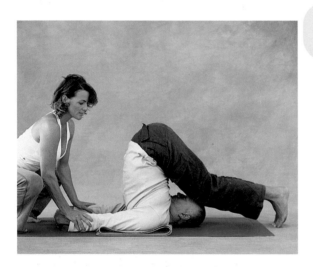

1 Lie on your back on a padded base. In order to maintain the natural cervical curve in the neck, raise the shoulders and upper back higher than the head, allowing space for the natural cervical curve to stay intact. On inhale, lift the feet off the floor. On exhale, gently swing the legs over the head into the plough pose (see also page 75). Support the back with both your hands, aiming to keep the shoulders and elbows in line. Alternatively, stretch out your arms and clasp your hands. A partner can help keep you aligned with your hips directly above your shoulders.

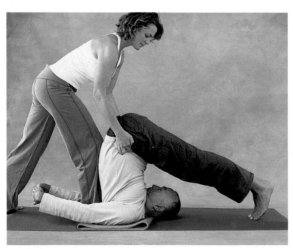

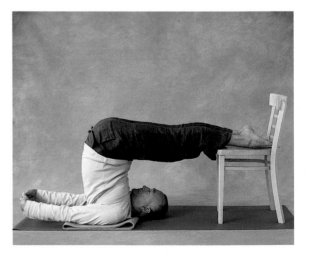

2 Inhale, straighten the spine and open the chest. Straighten your legs and press your toes into the mat, lifting the pubic bone up and away from the sternum to lengthen the pubic abdomen.

Modification: Alternatively, lower your feet onto a chair for the plough pose. Your hands can support your lower back or be clasped behind you, as shown here. This variation puts less strain on the back. Check that the neck is released and the jaw is not locked.

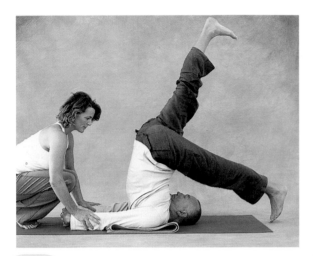

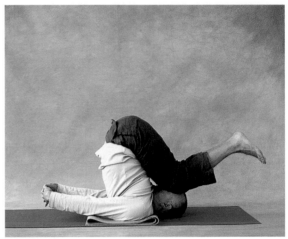

3 On inhale, lift your left leg to the vertical. On exhale, return to plough. Repeat with your right leg, alternating three times.

4 Gently uncurl your body, bending both of your knees to your head.

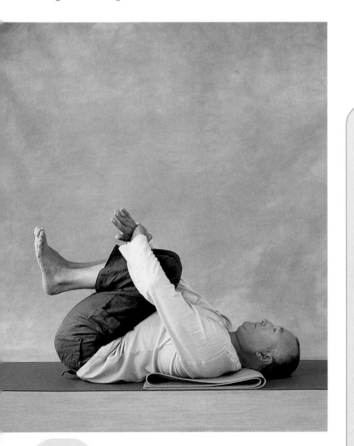

5 Hug your knees into your abdomen in apanasana, resting and breathing.

Advanced Plough Raises:
BENEFITS & EFFECTS

- The predominant effect of inversions on the cardio-vascular system is a complete reversal of the circulatory dynamics experienced by upright posture. In addition to the plough position demonstrated on these pages, see shoulderstand (sarvangasana, page 74) and headstand (sirsasana, pages 46–47) for correcting hypotension and varicose veins.

- Venous drainage of legs and abdomino-pelvic organs is greatly enhanced.

- Venous return to the heart is dramatically increased due to drainage of the blood reservoirs in the abdomen (liver, spleen and inferior vena cava), which stimulates the right atrial heart reflex and invigorates the pulmonary circulation.

- An initial increase in heart rate occurs. which is one reason why inversions are contraindicated in cases of medium-to-high blood pressure.

- Intracranial arterial pressure is significantly increased in a full inversion. Although beneficial to a healthy body, it is potentially dangerous in cases of hypertension.

- The carotid sinus reflex is activated and begins to slow down the heart rate and reduce blood pressure.

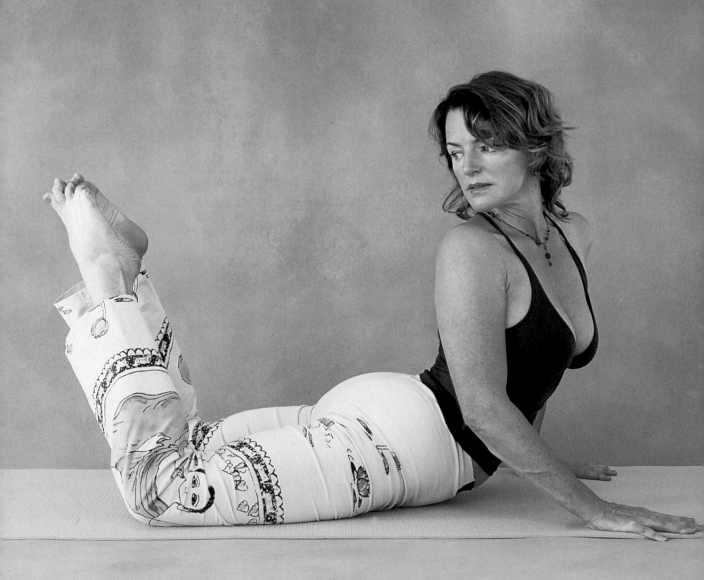

the digestive system:

the inner fire

A strong digestive fire is considered essential for good health. When this fire, known as agni, is impaired due to imbalance, the body's metabolism is affected. Undigested food (ama) may congest the large intestine, producing toxins that can bring about all sorts of disorders. Ayurveda suggests that the root of disease is due to the accumulation of ama and removing such stagnation from the intestines is crucial to maintaining health. A yogic method of cleansing the system, called nauli (a development of uddiyana bandha – see page 17) and a combination of yoga asanas, especially twists and backbends, will facilitate cleaning ama and energizing the intestines, so they will start to sing!

In most cases, indigestion is precipitated by tension, anxiety and frustration. It is therefore also important to digest emotionally, physically and mentally – to relax more and take plenty of time when eating. Make eating a sadhana (a yoga path), for we have to face it at least twice a day.

THE DIGESTIVE SYSTEM AND ORGANS

Essentially, digestion is the energy from food being made accessible to the body's cells. This happens via a process called catabolism, in which complex molecules are broken down into molecules small enough to be transported across cell membranes. The organs that play a role in this process constitute the digestive system, which is divided into two groups, the gastrointestinal tract and the 'accessory' organs.

The gastrointestinal tract is a continuous tube from the mouth to the anus. Its structures include the mouth, pharynx, oesophagus, stomach, and the small and large intestines. The lining of the gut tube has a mucous layer to allow absorption of nutrients and an outer layer of smooth muscle to perform the mechanical movements of digestion. The peritoneum is the two-layered internal lining of the abdominal cavity, which surrounds most of the abdominal organs, allows vessel and nerve transmission and helps stem infection and haemorrhage.

The accessory organs of digestion include the teeth, tongue, salivary glands, liver, gall bladder and pancreas, all of which have a role to play in the digestion process.

The **mouth** uses combined movement of the cheeks, tongue, teeth and jaw to carry out mechanical digestion, while saliva performs chemical digestion using enzymes.

The **oesophagus**, a muscular tube connecting the mouth to the stomach, uses muscular contractions (peristalsis) to push the food towards the stomach.

The **stomach** employs a churning, wave-like action to expose its contents to gastric juices, namely hydrochloric acid and pepsin, which breaks down proteins into smaller peptones. Once the food leaves the stomach it is in a liquid form known as chyme.

The **small intestine** is divided into three parts: duodenum, jejunum and ileum. The inner mucous membrane of the small intestine is highly adapted for digestion, and nearly all absorption of nutrients occurs here. Its glands produce useful enzymes and mucus, and the sheer length of the small intestine, as well as its folds and microvilli, provide a large surface area to optimize absorption. Mechanical digestion in the small intestine involves both segmentation and peristalsis. Segmentation is a circumferential contraction of alternate segments of the small intestine. Peristalsis propels the chyme onwards, although it is much weaker than oesophageal peristalsis.

On average, chyme remains in the small tract for three to five hours, giving time for the absorption of nutrients. Chemical digestion involves different enzymes for different food types.

- Carbohydrates are broken down into mono-saccharides and absorbed or used as blood glucose.
- Peptones are broken down into polypeptides and finally individual amino acids for absorption.
- Fats are broken down into short- and long-chain fatty acids and monoglycerides. Short-chain fatty acids are absorbed via the bloodstream, while long-chain fatty acids and monoglycerides are resynthesized into triglycerides and transported into the lymphatic system before finally arriving at the liver via the bloodstream.

The **large intestine** is subdivided into the caecum, colon, rectum and anal canal. Food moves first up through the ascending colon, then across the transverse colon, and next down through the descending portion before finishing in the sigmoid colon, which is continuous with the rectum. Three common sites of blockage are the ileo-caecal valve, right hepatic flexure (bend), the left splenic flexure and the sigmoid colon.

Taenia coli are longitudinal bands of muscle throughout the colon that give it a pouched appearance (haustra). Mechanical digestion involves haustral churning, peristalsis and mass peristalsis, the latter linked with defecation. Finally, some water, inorganic salts, epithelial cells, undigested food (usually fibre) and bacteria are eliminated as faeces.

The **liver** is situated below the diaphragm and to the right-hand side of the body. The liver has two lobes. These secrete bile salts (through hepatic ducts) into the common bile duct where it mixes with bile from the gallbladder. This is also joined by the pancreatic duct so that bile salts mix with pancreatic juice before being released into the duodenum. The main functions are the metabolism of carbohydrate, protein and fat; the synthesis of bile salts for digestion, and storage of vitamins (A, B12, D, E, K), minerals (iron and copper) and glycogen; the conversion of amino acids as required by the body; and the conversion of ammonia (the byproduct of protein catabolism) to urea for excretion in urine. In addition, it removes drugs, alcohol and hormones, and activates vitamin D.

The **gall bladder** is a long pear-shaped sac on the visceral surface of the liver. Hormonal stimulation activates the smooth muscle layer here to eject bile into the cystic duct. It stores and concentrates bile by absorbing water, secretes mucus to add to bile and ejects bile into the duodenum.

The pancreas is a gland below the liver. Islets of Langerhans (one per cent of pancreatic cells) form the endocrine portion of the gland, which secrete the hormones insulin and glucagons into the bloodstream to control glucose levels. Acini cells (the other 99 per cent of pancreatic cells) form the exocrine portion and secrete pancreatic juice for digestion. This juice contains water, salts, enzymes and sodium bicarbonate to buffer the acidic effect of pepsins from the stomach.

COMMON DIGESTIVE DISORDERS

Ulcers are crater-like structures that arise as a reaction to the acidity of gastric juice. This can occur in either the stomach (gastric ulcer) or, more commonly, the duodenum (duodenal ulcer). Ulcers are associated with anxiety, tension and the effects of prolonged arousal of the sympathetic nervous system. During sympathetic arousal, the secretion of mucus by glands in the gastro-intestinal tract – which form a protective lining against stomach acid – is inhibited, making the stomach and adjacent structures vulnerable. Other causes are smoking, coffee, excessive intake of fried and spicy foods and overuse of anti-inflammatory medication such as aspirin. Ulcers are usually painful soon after eating. The real danger is the risk of bleeding or perforation, which causes bacteria and food substances to leak into the peritoneal cavity causing peritonitis (inflammation of the peritoneum), a life-threatening condition.

Irritable Bowel Syndrome (IBS) is a common disruption of bowel function, mainly affecting the colon. Symptoms are either constipation, diarrhoea or alternating episodes of both. The most significant cause is stress, which prevents the parasympathetic system from functioning effectively during digestion. Food intolerances are also often to blame and may be reflected in episodic bloating of the bowel.

Inflammatory Bowel Disease (IBD) is not to be confused with IBS as it is much more serious. It can occur in two forms, both of which may involve intestinal bleeding: Crohn's disease and collitis. Crohn's disease is an inflammation of the gastrointestinal tract, anywhere along the route between the mouth and the anus. The most common region affected is the end of the small and/or beginning of the large intestine and the rectum. Ulcerative Collitis-Inflammation is restricted to the colon.

Diverticulitis is a disorder causing slight outpouchings of the wall of the colon. It may occur due to general overeating or the consumption of too much food that is high in animal protein and/or low in fibre. Poor mechanical digestion due to eating during periods of stress may also be a cause.

Indigestion occurs when your body is having difficulty fully digesting food and is most frequently experienced soon after eating. It may be a symptom of an underlying condition such as an ulcer. The usual cause, however, is overeating and/or eating foods not suited to your particular digestive system. Large amounts of fatty, fried or spicy foods are common culprits.

TREATMENTS AND THERAPIES

Orthodox medical treatments for digestive disorders include anti-inflammatory drugs, antacids and even steroids for extreme cases of IBD. The gradual introduction of the following yoga practices will also help heighten the performance of your digestive system. Do not, however, stop taking any drugs you have been prescribed without consulting your doctor first.

The asanas on the following pages, particularly twists and backbends, suggested will enhance the vayus – prana (inspiration), samana (assimilation) and apana (elimination); see page 12. Breathing practices (see pages 120–1) will energize, clear and soothe your system; yoga nidra (see page 123) will bathe the brain and facilitate ease throughout the entire body.

Other courses of action you can take to help your digestive system are:
- A 24-hour fast to clear your system. Consume only fresh juices and fruits. Do this on a rest day
- Improvements to your diet, ensuring it is balanced
- Washings (kriyas) and saltwater cleansings (see pages 21, 77 and 81)
- Practising uddiyana bandha – 'psychic suction' of the abdomen – and nauli (see page 77).

EATING MEDITATION

Tests carried out on rabbits found that while chewing grass, they were in a calm, meditative state due to the massaging effect that the chewing action has on the bony structures in the skull. To replicate this, take a five-minute breather before eating – this will allow the parasympathetic nervous system, which governs digestion, to prevail over the sympathetic. Chewing food slowly and thoroughly, like a cow chewing cud, will give time for emotional, mental and physical digestion.

Basic Supine Butterfly Twist

Suitable for all the disorders listed on pages 68–9, and a safe floor sequence for beginners, the butterfly twist works as a moving meditation on 'samana', the assimilating pranic pattern that facilitates digestion, by flowing in a continual vinyasa without pausing. Samana vayu, prana vayu and apana vayu (the eliminative, expulsive, detox pattern) are enhanced by this sequence of postures. This twist stretches the quadriceps, hamstrings, psoas and gluteal muscles, and stimulates the stomach meridian running through the centre of the body and into the abdomen.

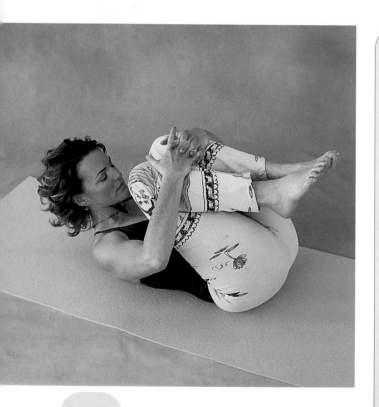

1 Lie on the floor in supine – facing up – position. Hug the thighs to the abdomen in apanasana (see also page 22) and squeeze on a deep outbreath. Release the legs on the inbreath. Relax the shoulders as you practise. Repeat for ten breaths. Focus on langhana, the long outbreath, to detoxify.

Basic Supine Butterfly Twist:
BENEFITS & EFFECTS:

- Apanasana (step 1) is the classic eliminative pose, encouraging general relaxation and detoxification. It is excellent for treating constipation and blockages in the gut.
- Butterfly-opening the hips and groins creates space and relaxation for abdominal organs and muscles.
- On inhalation, the openness of the abdomen facilitates the downwards descent of the diaphragm, which massages the abdominal viscera (abdominal organs).
- The twist action compresses the liver and ascending colon on the right side (when knees bend to the left), and compresses the stomach, spleen, pancreas and descending colon on the left side (when knees bend to the right). The piston-like action of the diaphragm thus rhythmically massages these organs in synchrony with the breath.
- Due to the twisting action, the alternate abdominal obliques are stretched, which improves the tone of the abdominal wall.
- The outstretched arms encourage deep yoga breathing, which facilitates digestion.

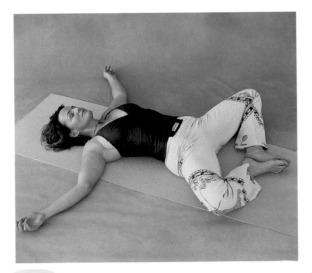

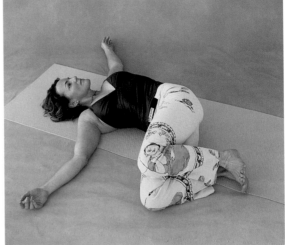

2 Now, with your knees bent, wing them open, like a butterfly, supta baddha konasana. Keep the soles of your feet together and your arms outstretched to the sides. Observe your breathing and maintain an open chest throughout for unrestricted breathing. On inhale, complete the yoga breath; on exhale, contract uddiyana and mula bandha as you drain your lungs.

3 On inhale, lift the left knee up. On exhale, lower the bent left leg to touch the right into a supine twist. Turn your face to the left, keeping the shoulders down towards the earth, the chest open and the arms outstretched for five breaths. To deepen the twist, tuck your knees closer to your right elbow.

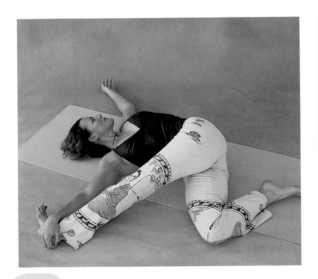

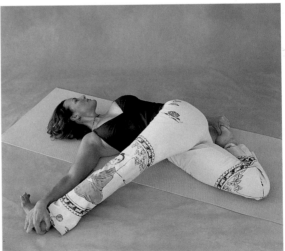

4 On inhale, straighten the top leg and catch the foot (or leg) with the opposite arm. This will intensify the squeezing action of the twist, stretching the back of the leg and buttock. Hold for five breaths.

Advanced option: Aim to catch the other foot of the bent leg with the free arm, so both feet are bound. Take five breaths, Inhale, return to butterfly pose (step 2). Exhale, relax. Repeat steps 3 and 4 on the other side.

Intermediate Cat to Hero

This sequence develops from cat, to twisting cobra, to the classic hero pose. Suitable for intermediate students, the postures can alleviate irritable bowel syndrome (IBS), inflammatory bowel disease (IBD), mild diverticulitis and indigestion. These postures are helpful in reducing obesity, by means of stretching and toning the abdominal area and reducing pranic blockages in the gut tube. If you have any serious back, knee or ankle problems, avoid twisting in cobra and hero. Sit on a block, ask an experienced instructor to check your alignment and omit the reclining hero pose. If doing this pose, however, tuck your tailbone under and release and lengthen your lower back. Do not practise uddiyana bandha when suffering from stomach ulcers, diarrhoea or acute IBD.

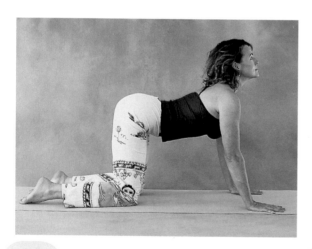

1 Begin in the tabletop, all-fours, position. Make sure the hands are directly beneath your shoulders and the knees are below your hips. Press the palms down to the floor, spreading your fingers out. On inhale, dip the spine like a snake, stretching the abdomen, chest and throat, and looking up. Lift your tailbone up as high as you can. Be sure not to crook your neck.

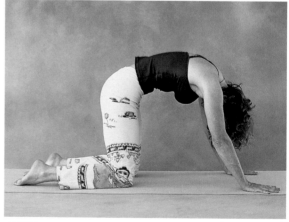

2 On exhale, arch your spine as high as you can, curling your chin towards your chest, tucking your tailbone under in the cat pose (bidalasana), contracting and hollowing uddiyana bandha (see page 17). Repeat steps 1 and 2 five times without strain. On the final spine dip, practise the lion pose (see page 119) to cleanse the tongue, looking up to your midbrow (shambhavi mudra, see page 122) and applying all three bandhas (tribandha, see pages 16–17). Hold momentarily, then release the locks and breath, dipping the spine again. Counterpose in extended child (see page 45), breathing into the abdomen.

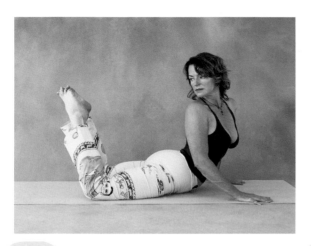

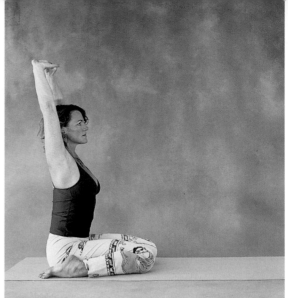

3 Inhale and swim the pelvis through the arms into baby cobra (see also page 100). If you experience any discomfort in the back, place the hands further forwards. Draw the shoulder blades down your back and hold for five breaths, maintaining symmetry on the left and right sides. Now lower the elbows to the floor, so the forearms run parallel in front of you. Breathe ten full breaths (great sphinx). Lift the arms so only your hands are on the floor (cobra), bend the knees to vertical and turn the head to one side, exhaling. Inhale, return to centre. Exhale, repeat with the head to the other side. Do this five times. Counterpose in downward dog or child's pose (see pages 40 and 45) to restore.

4 Now sit back in hero pose (seated vajrasana) by lifting to a kneeling position so that you are sitting your buttocks between your lower legs and your heels are pointing up on either side of your thighs. Raise the arms overhead and interlock the hands, palms facing upwards. Keeping the spine straight, stretch the entire abdominal cavity by applying a subtle uddiyana bandha for 20 breaths. Spread and root the tops of your toes.

Cat to Hero:
BENEFITS & EFFECTS:

- The cat pose alternately stretches and compresses the abdominal contents to cleanse and renew the blood reservoirs in the abdomen.
- Practising uddiyana bandha on outbreath further compresses the abdominal organs and the venous blood reservoirs, which flushes arterial blood into the abdominal area, vitalizing it.
- In the lion breath (simhasana), the act of stretching the tongue invigorates the upper digestive tract and cleanses the tongue, removing bad breath.
- The cobra has a massaging effect on the diaphragm due to the resistance exerted on the abdominal wall by the floor (the floor prevents the abdomen from distending). The twisting pattern of the head rotation focuses the effect on alternate sides of the abdomen.
- The hero pose (vajrasana) is considered the ultimate digestion posture, the only posture that can be practised directly after eating to reduce indigestion.
- The hero kneeling position limits circulation to and from the legs, thereby promoting blood flow to and from the digestive organs simultaneously stretching the entire abdominal region.
- The sequence stimulates samana vayu, the assimilating, balancing pranic pattern (see page 12).

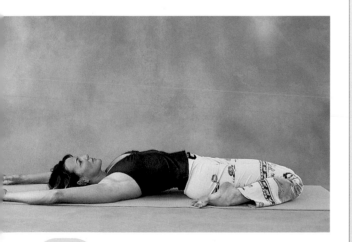

5 Exhale and lower your upper body towards the floor in a reclining hero pose (supta virasana) by first leaning back onto your hands, then your forearms, gradually coming all the way down. If necessary, lift your knees a little off the floor but do not allow the knees to be wider than your hips – this will cause strain on the hips and lower back. Hold for ten breaths. To come out, lift back into the hero pose.

Shoulderstand, Half Shoulderstand and Plough

A brilliant digestive posture, the shoulderstand is often described by Iyengar as the queen of all postures. Deeply restorative and healing, the topsy-turvy poses revive heart and brain and facilitate circulation. This sequence leads you through from full shoulderstand (sarvangasana) to half shoulderstand (vipareeta karani) to plough (halasana) to ear pressure pose (karnapidasana). Inversions calm and balance the neuroendocrine system as well as draining the abdominal organs.

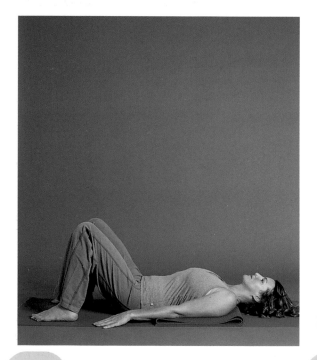

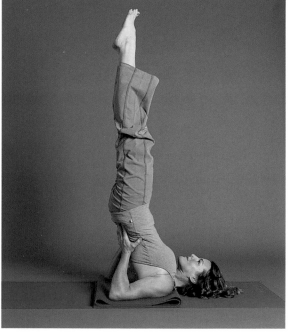

1 Lie semi-supine (with bent knees and the spine aligned) with the shoulders on a padded base (your head should be slightly lower to preserve cervical curve). Keep your arms by your sides, with the palms of the hands facing down.

2 On inhale, swing the legs up, bending the knees towards the brow. Raise your legs and back off the floor. Support the lower back firmly with your hands. Cup the kidneys, drawing the elbows in line with the shoulders. Straighten your legs and press them together. Relax the throat, jaw and face. Hold for 30 breaths and visualize the upper chakras (see pages 14–15).

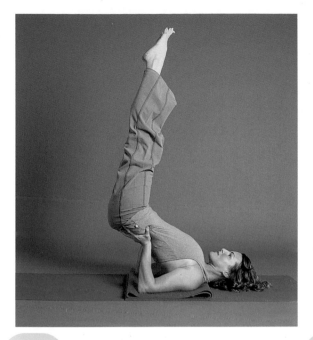

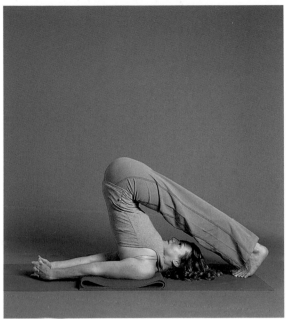

3 Lower the hips slowly, supporting the back by cupping the sacrum, and hold the half shoulderstand for 15 breaths, or as long as is comfortable. Keep the hips aligned, straighten the legs, look to your navel and move the chest and pubic bone away from each other.

4 Now lower your straight legs over your head into the plough position (see also pages 64–65). Your toes should be on the floor, or on a chair to modify. Straighten your arms in the opposite direction and interlock your fingers. Hold for ten breaths.

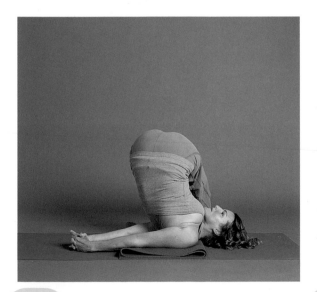

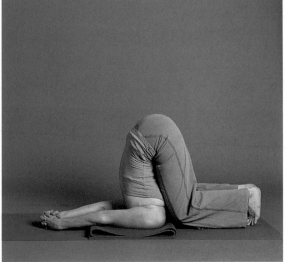

5 To intensify abdominal renewal, use your toes to walk your legs to your right side as far as possible without strain. Continue to face the sky and keep equal weight through both shoulders to maintain a firm foundation. Hold the twisting halasana for five breaths. Now walk over to the left side of the body to repeat.

6 Return the legs to plough and bend your knees in close to your head in ear pressure pose (karnapidasana). Aim to squeeze your ears with your knees, breathing into the kidney area. Avoid straining the neck. To modify, you can rest the knees towards the brow instead. Rest for ten breaths.

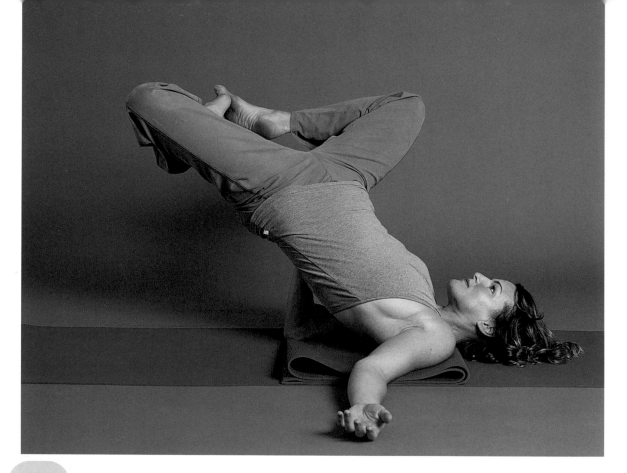

7 Now carefully lift your knees and support your lower back as if going into a shoulderstand again (step 2), but keep your knees bent. With the soles of the feet together (or set lotus posture for adepts), wing open your hips in a butterfly. Twist the pelvis to the right, cupping your sacrum with your right hand, and extend the left arm to the side, palm up. Hold for ten breaths and repeat to twist to the left.

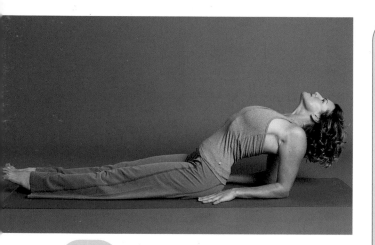

8 Lower your back and legs to the floor in supine corpse position for ten breaths. As a counterpose, move into fish pose (matsyasana). Lift your upper body to rest on your elbows, pressing your palms by your sides and letting your head drop back carefully. Lift your chest high towards the ceiling so that your back arches like a bridge, opening the back door to the heart. Hold for ten deep breaths then relax to the floor.

Shoulderstand
BENEFITS & EFFECTS:

- The half-shoulderstand pose, vipareeta karani, drains abdominal venous blood reservoirs (the spleen and liver), thereby stimulating the influx of arterial blood into the abdominal organs.
- The pose stimulates samana vayu (the flow of prana around the abdomen) and agni, the digestive fire, associated with the manipura chakra.
- The massaging effect of the diaphragm in steps 2–5 is enhanced by the application of uddiyana bandha (see page 17) and further stimulates the irrigation of the abdominal contents.
- Cleanses the lower abdominal organs and intestines, encouraging blood flow to the upper organs, chest and head to refresh the lungs, heart and brain.

Abdominal Massage
(Nauli)

This 'churning' massage is a development of uddiyana bandha (see page 17) and is an intermediate-to-advanced practice. Only embark on this breathing exercise once you have mastered uddiyana bandha and strengthened the rectis abdomini muscles. The massage isolates these muscles, using them as a churning rod to create a powerful belly massage.

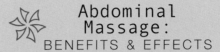

Abdominal Massage:
BENEFITS & EFFECTS

- Like a washing machine, the abdominal visceral are churned and the digestive tract squeezed with the use of the rectus abdomini (the long muscles that run vertically through the abdomen).
- Digestive ailments are removed, particularly constipation, acidity and bloating.
- A powerful, cleansing wave washes through the organs with the deep abdominal muscular toning, enhancing psycho-emotional digestion, balancing the prana patterns – the energy flow throughout the system – and connecting you to your roots.

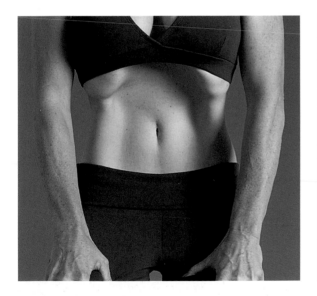

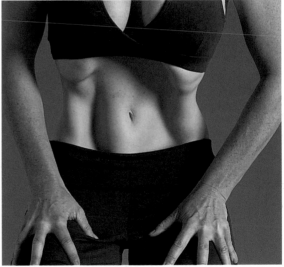

Stage one (uddiyana bandha): (Do not attempt during menstruation or pregnancy.) Stand with the feet apart, knees bent and hands on the thighs. Breathe in deeply. Empty the lungs through the mouth, retaining the outbreath through jalandhara bandha (see throat contraction on page 17). Suck in the rectus and transverse abdomini muscles to create a central concave curve. Hold for as long as possible, then release and inhale deeply. Relax. Repeat five times.

Option: As you breathe in, raise the arms skywards in a wide circle. Then, as you breathe out, draw the palms face down through the central front axis of the body.
Stage two (nauli): Once adept, try isolating the rectus abdomini and moving it to the right of the abdomen. Practise churning the muscles to the left (vama nauli) and to the right (dakshina nauli) three times each. Release and relax in a forward bend. Repeat five times, but do not repeat this practice within 24 hours.

Advanced Twisting Vinyasa

Suitable for all digestive disorders that are not in the acute stage. If you find the following sequence too demanding, practise the two twists given separately, following steps 1 and 3 three times each. To create a more challenging vinyasa, begin with five rounds of sun salutations (see pages 52–54); alternatively, begin with the archetypal spiral (see page 103).

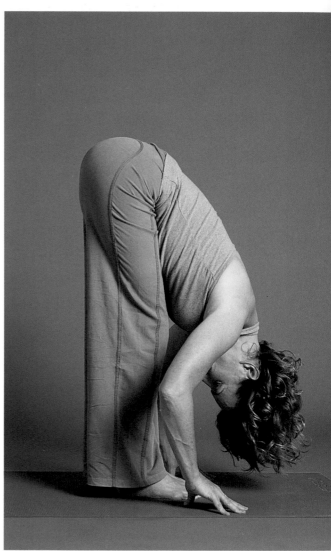

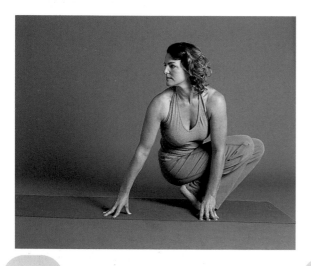

1 Bring the feet together. Squat on the balls of the feet, facing forwards with the spine straight. On inhale, lift your chest to lengthen your abdomen. On exhale, turn your upper body to the right, touching the fingers of both hands to the floor and turning the chin far to the right. Alternatively, place the right palm on the lower back, with the elbow pointing behind you. Use both arms as leverage to increase the rotation. Harness uddiyana bandha (see page 17) in the squatting twist for ten breaths. Repeat on the other side.

2 Now come up into a standing forward bend, uttanasana, with the feet planted on the ground. Draw the head towards the floor with the arms bent. Drop your heels into the ground and bend your knees as necessary to release your back. Lift the dome of the arches in your feet to cultivate a 'spring' in your step. Remain in position for ten breaths.

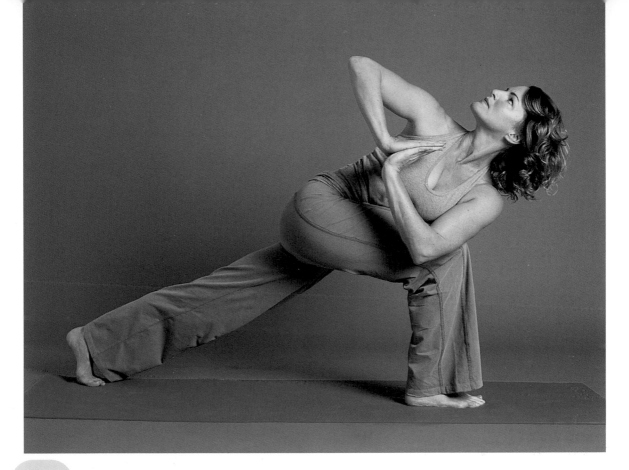

3 From the forward bend, move into the lunging twist (parsvakonasana). Glide the left leg back and bend the right knee into a lunge. On exhale, twist the upper body to the right, bringing the left elbow to the outside of the right thigh. Bring your palms together with bent elbows extending away from each other.

Your left upper arm rests on the outside of the right thigh and your right elbow points upwards. Broaden the collar bones, draw the scapulae down the back and look over the right shoulder. Take ten breaths. Inhale, return to the standing forward bend and repeat on the other side.

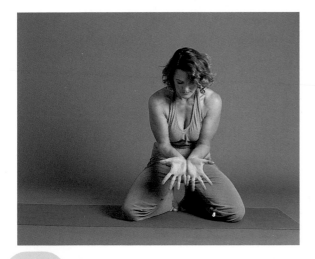

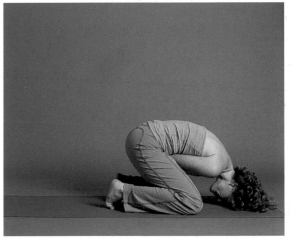

4 Now kneel with wide knees in preparation for the peacock pose (mayurasana). Kneel on the mat and place the outside edges of your hands together with the thumbs on the outside and pointing away from you and the fingers stretched out as far as you can.

With the fingers turned back towards your body, place your hands on the floor, between your knees, and bend your elbows towards your abdomen. Place your forehead on the mat, raise your hips and lean forwards to balance on your hands, brow, knees and toes.

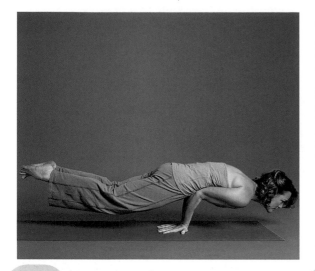

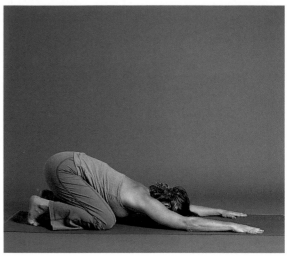

5 Gradually take the knees back into full peacock pose, mayurasana. Look to the floor and take five deep breaths, bending your elbows into your body. Stretch your legs out behind you, aiming to hold your body in a straight line. Balance and breathe.

6 Relax back into extended child's pose (see page 45) as a counterpose for 10–20 breaths, pressing the lengthened abdomen onto your thighs.

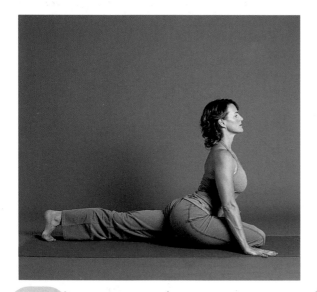

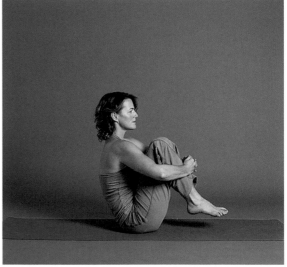

7 Slide your right leg forwards. Place your hands, palms flat, beside your knees, and keep your back toes tucked under. Your right knee should face forwards and diagonally to the right, and your right heel tucks to the left of your pubic bone. Straightening the back leg with the toes tucked under may intensify the asana. Lift your chest and head and press your shoulder blades downwards, lengthening your neck like a swan and looking up for five breaths. Repeat on the other side, linking the pose with downward dog.

8 Now slide the back leg forwards and sit back with bent knees, curling into the 'cosmic egg'. Wrap your arms around your shins, balancing on the sitting bones and breathe for five to ten breaths. Focus on the outbreath, cultivating mula and uddiyana bandhas (see pages 16–17) to enhance prana and apana.

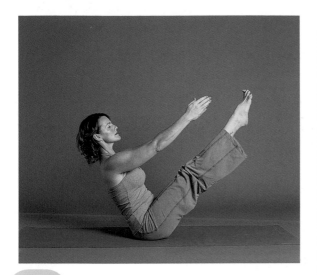

9 Now move into the boat pose, navasana. On inhale, lift the sternum skywards to straighten the spine, leaning back. Exhale, broaden the collar bones, lift the front of the armpits and stretch the arms towards the toes. Aim to straighten the legs, creating a 'v' shape with the body. If this is too intense, bend the knees, bringing the shins parallel to the floor in half boat. Hold for five to ten breaths. Alternate the boat and egg (steps 8 and 9) three to five times, inhaling to boat and exhaling to cosmic egg.

Twisting Vinyasa: BENEFITS & EFFECTS

- The squatting stance reduces blood flow to the legs, allowing greater circulation to the abdomen, oxygenating the organs and facilitating waste removal.
- Squats and twists combined with uddiyana bandha practice (see page 17) compress the internal organs, which are rhythmically massaged by the descent of the diaphragm. The diaphragm descends like a parachute.
- Both the intense forward bend (uttanasana) and downward dog are forward flexions, which drain venous blood from the abdominal organs and refresh the brain.
- Asymmetrical hip-opening postures, as shown in step 7, energize the colon on the side of the leg that is stretched back to relieve tension or blockages.
- The cosmic egg deepens apana vayu, the eliminative pattern (see page 12), relaxing and detoxing the body.
- The boat pose squeezes the abdominal organs by engaging the abdominal wall, pelvic diaphragm and respiratory diaphragm, strengthening the body's core.

Air Cleansing
(Swana pranayama)

This can be practised to revitalize and reoxygenate the digestive system, and is especially beneficial for getting rid of stale air, reducing gas and constipation, toning the digestive organs and stimulating the appetite (stoking the agni). Do not practise this if you suffer from heart conditions, stomach ulcers, an overactive thyroid or diarrhoea.

1 Sit in a comfortable position, or simple kneeling, with the knees wide apart and both hands on top of them. Breathe in deeply, then exhale and empty the lungs as fully as you can. Lean forwards, pressing the hands on the knees, and stick out the tongue (like in lion pose on page 119). Breathe in and out as if panting, simultaneously expanding (on inhalation) and contracting (on exhalation) the abdomen for 20 breaths. Do not strain.

2 For an advanced method, practise in the same way but retain the outbreath. This is called agnisar kriya or vahnisara dhauti.

Digestive Cleansing

This series of exercises forms an accompaniment to the abdominal massage described on page 77, yet doing it on its own will reinvigorate the digestive system. It is suitable for all, but should be practised very gently if you have an ulcer or other similar condition. Try to spread the work of the stretch throughout the body.

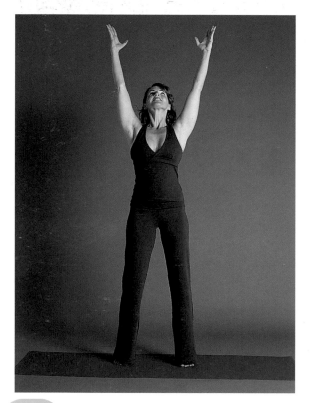

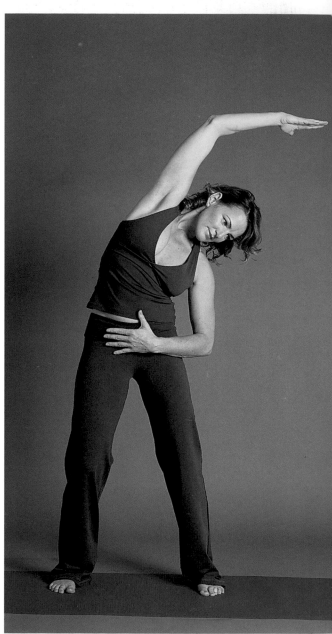

1 Stand in raised mountain pose, tadasana, with the feet slightly apart. Inhale, raise the arms overhead, and turn the palms towards each other. Imagine a positive energy charge coming into your body. Extend upwards, raising onto the tiptoes. Look straight ahead and hold for five breaths. On exhale, release to standing and lower the arms to the sides.

2 Arch laterally into swaying mountain pose, tiryaka tadasana. Place your feet hip-width apart and raise your right arm overhead. Rest your left hand on your lower abdomen. On exhale, lean to the right, circling the arm over the head, retaining the outbreath for a few moments and looking down to release the neck. Inhale, return to centre and repeat on the other side.

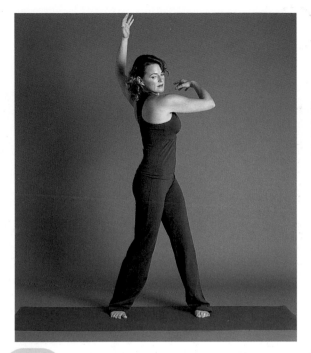

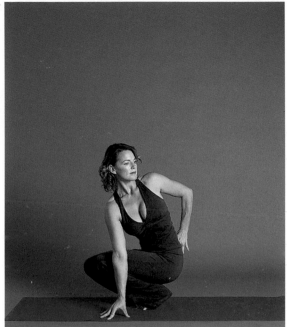

3 Return to mountain pose before moving into a waist rotation, kati chakrasana. On inhale, raise the arms out to the sides at shoulder level. On exhale, twist to the left, bringing the right hand to the left shoulder, the left hand behind you to the left side, and the chin to the right shoulder. Hold the outbreath, to enhance the twist action. Inhale, return to centre and repeat on the other side (swing rhythmically).

4 Squatting twist: Squat with feet together and draw the right arm outside the left thigh, twisting to the left to massage the abdomen. Place your right hand on the floor beside the left foot and your left hand on the sacrum, the body's centre of gravity. Remain here for five breaths before repeating on the opposite side.

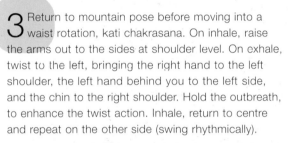

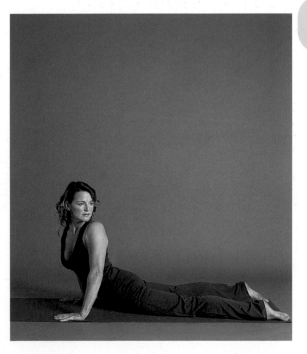

5 Twisting cobra (tiryaka bhujangasana): Lie face down in a supine prone position. Place the feet hip-width apart with the tops of the toes spread and pointing away from you. Now place the hands under the shoulders and on inhale, arch the spine. On exhale, twist the head and upper body to the left, looking to the heel of the left foot, diagonally stretching the abdomen (allow the elbows to bend slightly). Now twist to the right side. Inhale as you move and exhale as you twist, keeping the knuckle roots planted firmly into the floor and drawing the chest through the gateway of the arms.

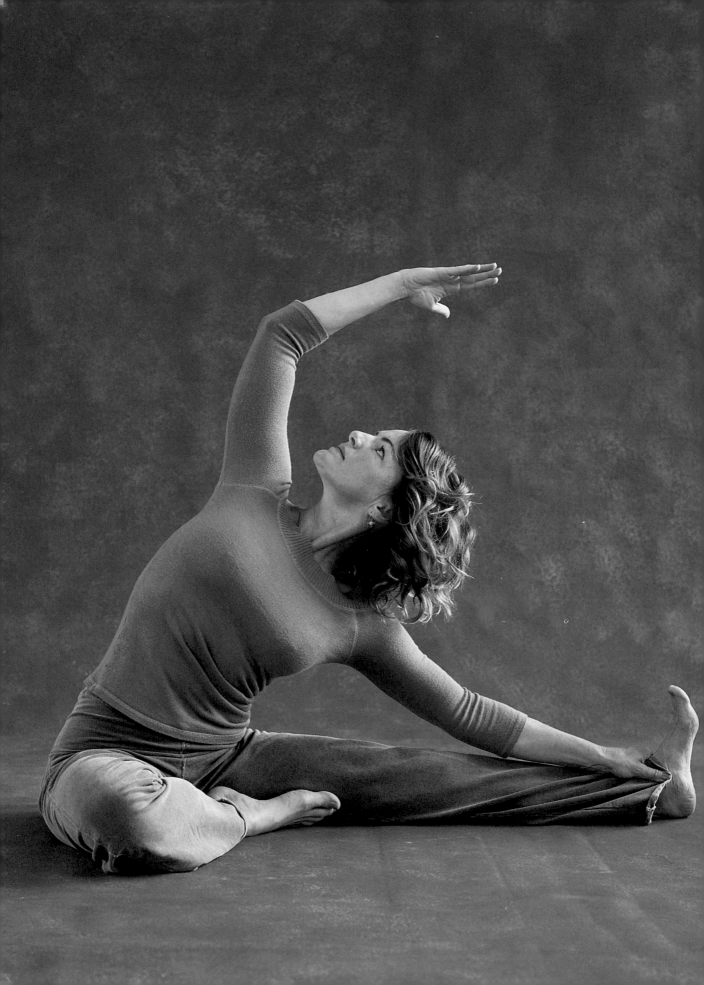

the genito-urinary system:

flow like water

The urogenital organs comprise a plumbing system with the dual function of reproduction and ridding the body of waste products in the form of urine. In the yogic view, the urogenital system is connected with the second chakra, swadhisthana ('one's own abode'), relating to the fulfilment of subconscious desires, sexual and creative expression, instinct and passions, and is linked with the fluid element of water. The two lower chakras, earth and water – instinct, sexuality – form the muddy ground of our humanity, and the springboard for evolution. Repressed or addictive fixations in these areas may hold us back, due to deep-seated impressions (habitual tendencies) of guilt, fear or inadequacy, in this complex psycho-emotional root.

It is essential to maintain the flow of pranic and psychic energy to the urogenital organs, for the koshas (sheaths) to be nourished – pranayama (energy sheath) and manomaya (mental sheath). A combination of restorative asanas, breathing, mudras, sankalpa, relaxation, meditation, and particularly long holds in restorative postures will engender healing.

THE URINARY SYSTEM

The efficient functioning of the urinary system is vital as it maintains the electrolyte–water balance of the fluids that bathe the body's tissue in a salty, aqueous environment. Other essential tasks include the regulation of blood volume and blood concentration by removing and collecting varying amounts of water and solutes. The urinary system is composed of the kidneys, ureters, bladder and urethra.

The kidneys are situated on either side of the lower spinal column and are suspended by their own blood vessels and renal fascia behind the peritoneal cavity. They are partially protected by the floating ribs and cushioned in an adipose (fatty) capsule. The right kidney is slightly lower than the left due to a degree of displacement by the liver.

The kidneys consist of an outer reddish region called the cortex and an inner brownish region known as the medulla. The functional unit is the nephron, a complex tube designed to allow maximum space for the filtration, reabsorption and secretion of nutrients. A nephron has two key components: the glomerulus – a tuft of capillaries – and an enveloping glomerular capsule, which is part of the renal tubule. This is the area where water and small solutes are filtered from the plasma of the bloodstream into the renal tubule. As the filtrate passes along the convoluted tubules, certain substances are reabsorbed or secreted. Ninety-nine per cent of the filtrate is reabsorbed, with only one per cent leaving the body.

Kidneys have to work extremely hard to allow a relatively small but vital excretion of waste via urine. Approximately 25 per cent of cardiac output is therefore directed to the kidneys via the renal arteries, resulting in the entire body's volume of blood being filtered about 60 times per day!

This reabsorption involves taking useful substances – such as water, glucose, amino acids and ions like sodium, potassium, chlorine, bicarbonate and phosphate – from the filtrate back into the blood. Meanwhile, tubular secretion takes other substances from the venous blood into the filtrate. This process of differential reabsorption and secretion maintains the body's acid/base balance (pH), as well as creating the byproduct urine.

By adjusting the proportion of sodium and potassium ions retained in the filtrate, the kidneys also play a key role in regulating blood pressure.

In cases of diabetes, hypertension and arteriosclerosis (see page 51) the micro-arteries of the renal circulation are among the first to suffer, resulting in disturbance of kidney function. Stress is another factor that has a huge impact on the urinary system. It causes an increase in the breakdown of protein and fats, resulting in increased strain on the kidneys to remove waste substances: urea and ammonia (byproducts of protein breakdown) and ketone bodies (byproducts of excessive fat metabolism).

The ureters transport urine from the kidney to the bladder, which lies just behind the pubic symphysis (the joint in front of the pelvis). An accumulation of urine stimulates stretch receptors in the smooth muscle of the bladder wall, which then contracts under the influence of parasympathetic nerve impulses. A coordinated relaxation of the internal bladder sphincter then permits passage of the urine into the urethra, a narrow tube running from the floor of the urinary bladder to the external environment. This process is known as micturition.

THE REPRODUCTIVE SYSTEM

The gonads, the primordia of the adult sex glands, appear in the fifth week of intrauterine life. The presence of a gene on the Y chromosome (for men) stimulates the gonads to develop into testes, which exit the body via the inguinal canal just before birth. In the absence of this canal (in women), the gonads become ovaries.

The uterus and vagina are formed from the fusion of the ducts that become the left and right Fallopian tubes, each associated with its own ovary. A similar tubular system in the male develops into the spermatic duct. The appearance of external genitalia also differentiates at the same time – from a common genital tubercle (elevation), which either forms a clitoris and vagina, or elongates into a penis.

Male sexual maturity is stimulated by increased production of the hormone testosterone at puberty, beginning the production of mature sperm cells, which can continue for most of adult life. In the female, however, all the eggs for life are produced during fetal life. The sexual maturity of the female is then achieved through a complex interaction of hormones beginning at puberty, which activates a few 'dormant' eggs each month. Only one monthly egg cell fully matures (ovulation). However, unless fertilized, the process of menstruation simply sheds the endometrium (womb lining) to prepare for the next menstrual cycle.

COMMON GENITOURINARY DISORDERS

Nephritis is employed here as a general term to cover the complex range of kidney disorders that involve inflammation, infection or both. Possible causes of such complaints include an ascending infection from the pelvis, prostatic obstruction, obstruction by a kidney stone, excess animal protein in the diet, drug-related problems or diabetes.

Cystitis and urethritis are similarly due to infection or inflammation, but this time of the bladder and/or urethra. The main symptom is pain on urination; cloudy urine usually indicates an infection. Possible causes include excessive consumption of alcohol, an overly acidic or sugary diet, long-term use of the contraceptive Pill and the e. coli infection.

Prostate problems are most commonly caused by an enlargement of the prostate – known as benign prostatic hypertrophy – which constricts urinary flow, making complete voiding difficult, and an infection known as prostatitis, which can give pain on urination and orgasm, and create an increased desire to urinate. The prostate gland is a small, walnut-shaped gland, which secretes fluid that contributes to sperm. It is located just below the bladder and encircles the urethra at this point.

Enlargement can be caused by acidic foods, a nutritional deficiency, poor abdominal tone, sluggish bowel, poor blood flow, sedentary occupation and lack of exercise. Any obstruction to the flow of urine caused by prostatic disorders can cause infections in the bladder, ureter and kidneys. Prostasis can be caused by infection elsewhere in the body, poor abdominal/pelvic floor tone or a general lack of exercise. Poor nutrition with acidic residue, and specifically a lack of zinc and essential fatty acids (EFAs), can also be a major factor.

Endometriosis is defined as growth of endometrial tissue (womb lining) outside the uterus. The tissue 'escapes' via the Fallopian tubes to areas as diverse as the kidney, bladder and sigmoid colon, or to more common places such as the ovaries and Fallopian tubes themselves. The pain associated with endometriosis is due to tissue migrating at the same time, or prior, to menstruation.

Male and female infertility is recognized as a problem when conception has not occurred despite over a year of trying. In the female it is usually due to blocked Fallopian tubes or a failure to ovulate in the first place. Common causes are pelvic inflammatory disease (PID), long-term use of the Pill, ovarian cysts, endometriosis, stress or excessive exercise. Male infertility, which tends to be the problem in 40 per cent of failures to conceive, can be as a result of smoking, taking anabolic steroids, excessive alcohol or caffeine, drinking oestrogen-contaminated water, or natural reasons like low sperm count. Difficulty in achieving or maintaining an erection can also play a role. Male impotence is usually due to psychological factors such as stress or worry about sexual performance, although it can also be secondary to loss of libido due to prostate problems.

THERAPIES AND TREATMENTS

Orthodox medical treatments for the common disorders discussed vary greatly, from hormone therapy or surgery for endometriosis to Viagra for impotence (although not recommended for people with a heart or liver condition) through to antibiotics for urinary infections and hormonal therapy or drugs for infertility.

You can also help yourself by integrating yogic practices, and variable combinations of bandha, mudra, asana, pranayama, meditation and deep relaxation, into your daily life. Although certain practices are recommended for particular disorders here, the suggestions given, especially the pelvic floor exercises and bandhas, constitute a general programme. Please note that the possibility of cancer should always be ruled out before commencing with any self-help for prostate problems.

Vajroli mudra (see pages 16 and 89) is considered a powerful yogic tool to overcome genitourinary disorders. This practice involves the conscious contraction of the whole urogenital apparatus and is said to lead to mastery over instinctive life: an ability to harness and sublimate our base energy toward a higher purpose.

Another straightforward form of self-treatment is simply to reassess your diet. A day or two of consuming only juices and infusions can be helpful in acute cases to flush out the system before rebuilding it. Cranberry, watermelon juice and parsley tea are particularly good. Increasing your intake of fresh fruit and vegetables, whole grains and essential fatty acids can also be hugely beneficial – especially for kidney, bladder and urethra inflammation or infections. An increase in essential fatty acids, as well as zinc, is also extremely useful for prostate problems. These fats can be found in sunflower seeds, sesame seeds and fish oils, while zinc can be obtained from the consumption of brown rice, eggs, pumpkin seeds, nuts and wheatgerm. Often overlooked, the importance of drinking plenty of water should also be remembered, especially in cases of infection.

Ashwini Mudra

This mudra, meaning 'horse gesture', contracts the anal sphincter muscle region in order to improve tone and function of the underlying muscles. The contractions have the effect of squeezing the pelvic organs rhythmically, improving blood flow to the area, which nourishes, purifies and heals. The apanic pattern (detoxification; see vayus on page 12) is drawn upwards, creating energetic lift. This practice is suitable for pre- and postnatal care, recovering haemorrhoids, male prostate disorders and general confidence-building. Here, we combine the pelvic lift with an inner muscular contraction of the anal sphincter muscle. According to the classic Hatha yoga text, the *Gheranda Samhita*, 'This ashwini is a great mudra; it gives strength and vigour, and prevents premature death'. Do not practise this, however, if you suffer from high blood pressure, haemorrhoids or anal fistula.

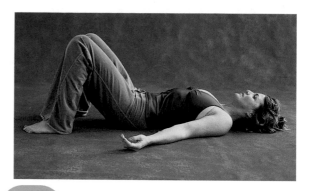

1 Lie semi-supine, with knees raised and arms out to the sides. Practise the complete ujjayi breath (see page 120). As you exhale, begin to cultivate uddiyana and mula bandhas (see pages 16–17) so that, at the end of exhalation, they are deeply engaged. Repeat the cycle, inhaling the complete yoga breath.

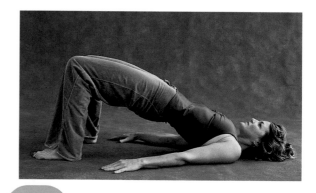

2 On inhale, press your feet and arms into the floor and lift your pelvis upward into the bridge pose, peeling the spine away from the floor. Keep your knees and feet parallel and your knees over your heels, but direct them away from the hips, in line with the toes. Slowly contract and dilate the anal aperture, as if to withhold bowel movement, ten times. Hold each contraction for a few seconds. On exhale, relax, lowering your pelvis to the floor to come out of the posture. Repeat the isolated movement rhythmically for ten rounds, keeping the rest of the body relaxed, including the other genitourinary muscles, if possible.

Advanced option: Hold the breath (breath retention) while performing the sphincter contraction. Repeat the sequence for up to 25 rounds.

Seated Mudra

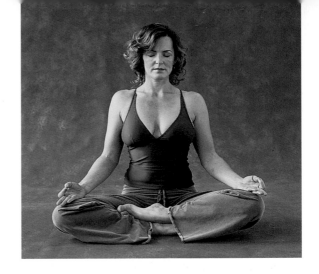

This pelvic-floor (Kegel) exercise (ashwini-mula-vajroli) helps to differentiate, isolate and strengthen the various muscle beds in the pelvic floor. It is invigorating for the whole pelvic floor and is useful for preventing or correcting incontinence, prostate problems, and can be done pre- or postnatally.

1 Sit with both legs outstretched. Cross the left leg so that the sole of the foot presses the inner right thigh. For men, press the left heel into the perineum. For women, the left heel should press the vagina. Place the right foot on top of the left calf, pressing the right heel directly on the pelvic bone, above the genitals (the right heel should be directly above the left heel). This is siddhasana, the practise seal for mudras and pranayamas. Feel as if you are planted into the ground, aware of the four bony roots of your pelvis dropping earthwards: the two sitbones, pubic bone and tailbone.

2 Now concentrate on the region of muladhara chakra (see page 14). Straighten the spine and rest the hands on the knees. Draw your focus to the pelvic floor and practise ashwini mudra (anal contraction) ten times (see above), rapidly and rhythmically. Now move your awareness to mula bandha (cervix or root of penis – see page 16) and repeat the contraction ten times; notice it is more subtle than the anal contraction. Now draw your awareness to vajroli mudra at the front of the pelvic floor genitourinary muscle, and repeat the contraction ten times.

3 Repeat the sequence, synchronized with the breath: on inhale, contract, hold your breath and lift; on exhale, release. Repeat five times at all three sites.

4 To finish, relax and focus on the chidakash, the mind space just in front of the closed eyes, recalling any different sensations with detachment.

Lizard Mudra

This practice helps problems linked to the pelvic floor, including sexual vitality, prostate function, infertility and menstrual discomfort. It is also therapeutic for backache and asthma.

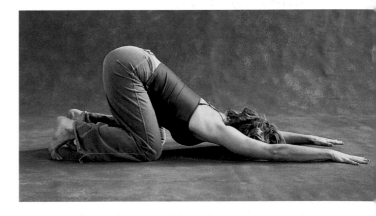

1 Adopt the lizard, or crouching tiger pose by kneeling on your heels. Now raise your hips and lean forwards, so your knees are hip-width apart and the chest dips towards the floor with the chin resting towards the floor and the toes tucked under. Draw the arms in front of you in a passive backbend stretch with the palms flat on the floor. Stretch through the torso.

2 Practise mula bandha (see page 16). Bring your awareness to the perineum and gently contract the pelvic floor muscles ten times as you breathe.

3 Return to sitting and practise vajroli mudra (see page 16). Concentrating on the front genitourinary muscles, contract ten times, as if withholding urination.

Supported Half Shoulderstand to Butterfly

For the following exercise you will need a bolster or one or two firm pillows to elevate and support your pelvis against the wall. This will enable you to lift your lower body comfortably, retain the inverted posture for some time and relax in it for three to five minutes. The half shoulderstand, vipareeta karani, is good for prolapse, as it allows the uterus to find its correct position in the pelvic cavity, while the butterfly pose, baddha konasana, stimulates the ovaries, prostate gland, bladder and kidneys, encouraging cleansing. Regular practice of the butterfly until late pregnancy can help ease childbirth. Practise three times a day for ten minutes if possible. Do not practise inversions during menstruation.

Vipareeta Karani to Butterfly: BENEFITS & EFFECTS

- The inversion drains venous blood from the abdomino-pelvic organs and reduces the strain of gravity on the kidneys, which can be prone to dropping beneath the ribs.
- Using a bolster encourages deeper relaxation and better venous/lymphatic drainage.
- The butterfly releases tension in the lower abdomen and creates space for increased blood flow.

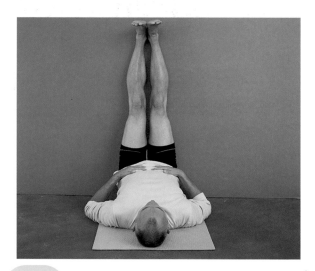

1 Position a bolster against the wall. Lie with the pelvis on the bolster and with the legs up the wall in a supported half shoulderstand. Keep your legs together and hands resting on the abdomen, palms down. Practise complete yoga breathing, concentrating your breath at the navel centre. Hold the posture for five to ten minutes, or for as long as comfortable.

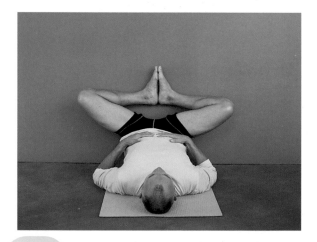

2 **Variation:** On exhale, bend your knees, draw your heels towards your pelvis and drop your knees to the sides in butterfly pose (supta baddha konasana). Press the soles of your feet together and aim to draw your knees towards the wall. Hold for one to three minutes, concentrating awareness at the navel centre.

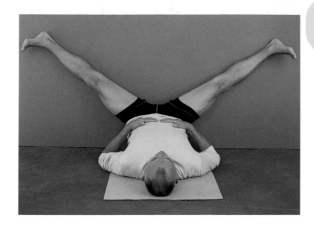

3 Now draw your legs up and out to the sides in the reclining angle pose, supta konasana, with flexed feet. Widen your legs as far as you can comfortably and engage the leg muscles. Aim to press the backs of the legs against the wall to deepen the stretch and pull up the inner thighs and quadriceps. Hold for two minutes, practising breathing into the belly. Relax and broaden the shoulders without straining your neck.

Seated Vinyasa

The seated twist, bharadvajasana, invigorates the spine and massages the abdominal organs. In this sequence, hip-opening is combined with twists to cleanse the lower abdomen and urogenital region. Focus on the triaxes of the vertical spine, the horizontal pelvis and the broad shoulder girdle.

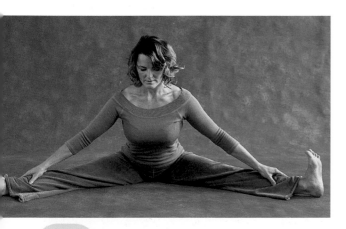

1 To begin, sit in seated staff (dandasana) with your legs out straight in front of you. On inhale, open the legs, rotating your thighs outward so the knees point upwards and feet are flexed (upavistha konasana). Place your hands below the knees and widen the legs as far as you can, stretching from the roots of the hamstrings at the hips and lengthening the back as you reach in a forward stretch. Hold for ten breaths, lifting the sternum with each inbreath to open the abdomen and chest. On inhale, lift the upper body, raising the arms to the sky. On exhale, fold into a forward bend. Hold for ten breaths.

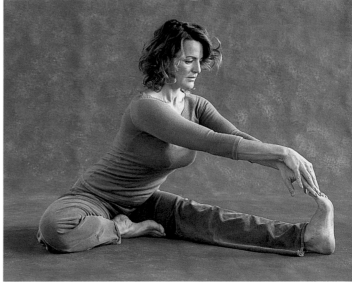

2 On inhale, return to the seated staff. Bend the right knee, bringing the right heel to the groin, and lean over the left knee to prepare for step 3 (janu sirsasana, head to knee posture). On inhale, lift the chest and stretch both sides of the trunk. On exhale, reach for the toes of the left foot with both hands. Hold for 20 breaths.

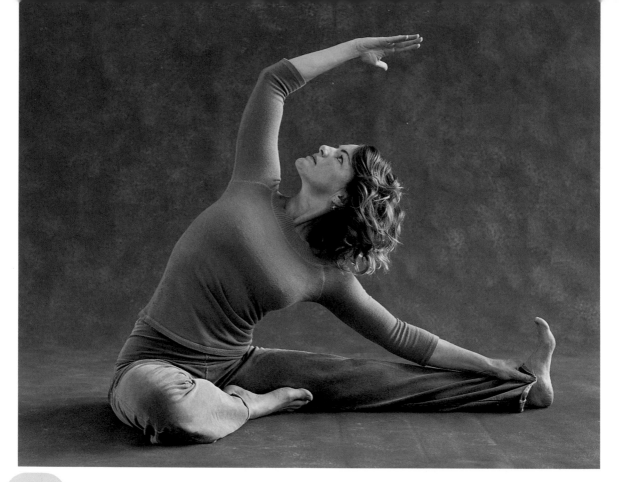

3 As you inhale, return to seated stance. Now turn the upper body so that the left side is in line with the left leg. On exhale, arch the trunk laterally over the left leg, drawing the right shoulder back. Arch the right arm over the head and follow with your head so that you are now looking towards your raised right hand. Slide your left hand towards your left ankle and anchor your right sitting bone so you do not tip your pelvis to one side. Hold for ten or more breaths. Return to face directly over the straight leg for ten more breaths, lifting and pressing down the right kidney with each outbreath.

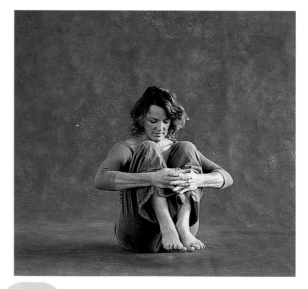

Seated Vinyasa:
BENEFITS & EFFECTS

- Janu sirsasana, the head-to-knee pose, creates space for the kidneys by stretching the overlying muscles of the back. It also stretches the spine, shoulders, hamstrings and groin.
- Hip-opening twists cleanse the pelvic region.
- To avoid slumping, rock forwards towards the front of your sitting bones while maintaining the back of the pelvis throughout the twist sequence.

4 Now bend both knees and bring them to your chest into the cosmic egg (see also page 80). Wrap your arms around the shins and balance on your sitting bones with your heels off the floor. Breathe until you feel restored and eased. This is a release pose that can be placed between difficult sequences to soothe the lower back and kidney area. Now repeat steps 1–4 with the right leg outstretched.

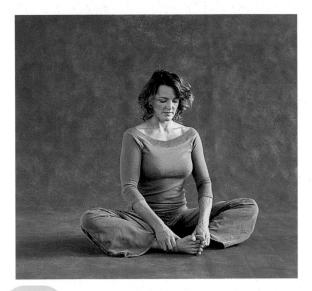

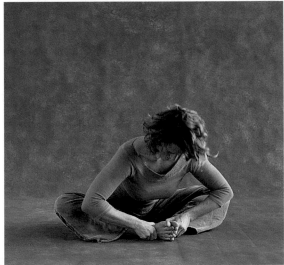

5 Seated with a straight spine, bend the knees and press the soles of the feet together in the butterfly pose (baddha konasana). Inhale in ujjayi pranayama (see page 120), exhale and drain the lungs deeply. Lift the pelvic floor, hollow the lower belly and tuck the chin towards the chest. Hold for ten breaths.

Now bend your elbows to draw your upper body towards the feet in a forward bend. Lift your kidneys with each inbreath and direct the breath there. Press your elbows to your knees and deepen the posture in a pose of humility for ten breaths. Release and move to step 6, or the advanced option below.

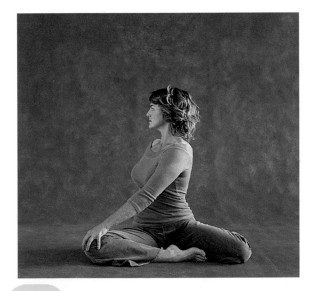

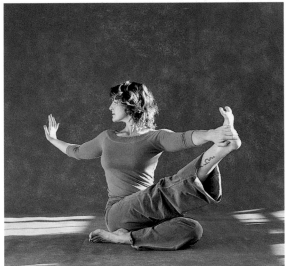

6 Inhale and carefully return to the butterfly with a straight back (step 5). Tuck your left lower leg back, so the left heel touches the outer left hip in a seated spinal twist (bharadvajasana). Aim to anchor both sitting bones. Placing the left hand on the right thigh and the right hand on the floor behind you, twist the trunk to the right. Lift the kidneys as you inhale and stretch, and twist as you exhale. Repeat for ten breaths. Return to butterfly pose. Repeat steps 5–6 on the other side.

Advanced option: For a further stretch and massage in the abdominal region, and following from step 5, lift and straighten your right leg, holding your right ankle with your left hand, stretching it out straight in front of you. Keep the opposite twist in the upper body, with your right arm stretched behind you and look toward your right hand. Your left knee should be tucked beneath you. Hold for ten breaths, and then release and repeat on the other side.

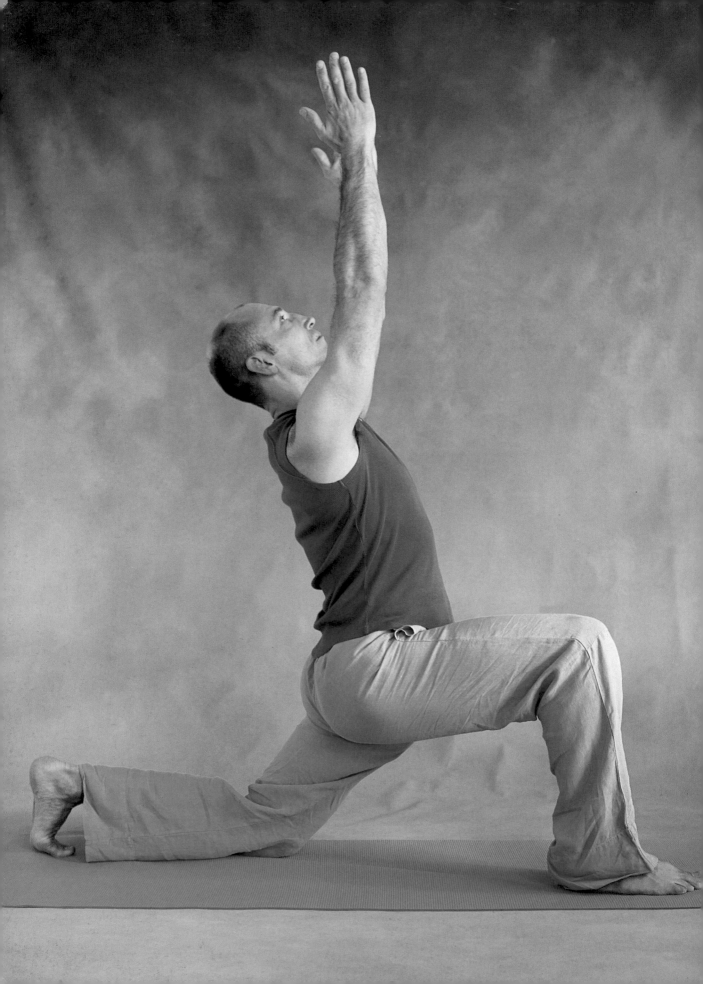

the spine:

the stem of intelligence

The spine is the brain's highly complex messaging system to the rest of the body, and the central highway to the brain. A healthy, integrated spine moves with ease and is not fractured, supporting us from behind, rooting us to earth through the tailbone (muladhara), and aspiring upward through the crown of the head. When people become disassociated from themselves, they may be described as having no backbone – being 'spineless'. A disjointed spine may show the attitude of straining forward into the future (jutting the chin forward) or fearfully falling back into the past (hunched shoulders, bowed thorax).

When we fold into forward bends, we bow to the unknown, the mystical, releasing the head to nourish parasympathetic nerve clusters housed in the brainstem and sacral region. This cranial-sacral connection activates calm. We yield by bending the knees. We practise backbends to celebrate life and welcome fresh inspiration. If we lock or tense during practice, we block the pulse of life moving through us.

The spine houses the chakras. We need to be anchored to live in the world, earthed through the tailbone. From this root, we spiral upward through the psychic centres towards transcendence.

THE DEVELOPMENT OF THE SPINE

The development of human embryos follows a specific and systematic process, shared by all vertebrates and known as a 'body plan'. Early shaping of the vertebrate body is accomplished by highly complex mass cell movements known as gastrulation, which create a three-layered 'sandwich' of embryonic cells: the primordial skin and nervous tissue on the outside and the gut tissue on the inside. Still a flat disc, the embryo folds from both head to tail and from left to right, the latter bestowing bilateral symmetry – the hallmark of a vertebrate.

Folding from head to tail creates a crescent moon shape around the umbilical cord, thereby establishing the primary spinal curve. The early vertebral column is initially one continuous mass of tissue, which then segments into discrete blocks known as somites, which eventually form vertebrae. This segmentation not only permits articulation of the vertebral column but also allows the spinal nerves to sprout from the now encased spinal cord toward specific structures relating to that segment.

At full-term the fetus is competing for space with the maternal abdominal organs and is neatly folded with arms and legs crossed in front of the body, a symbolic posture often assumed towards the end of yoga classes, suggesting a return to new life and renewal.

After birth, the secondary spinal curves in the cervical and lumbar region begin to develop. The cervical curve forms in response to the rapid development of the sense organs, whereas the stimulus for lumbar curve development is the vitally important crawling movements performed in the early struggle for independent activity. Increasing complexity of movement patterns becomes possible as the nervous system becomes more efficient and integrated, culminating in the triumph of the human species – balancing on two legs and walking.

ANATOMY OF THE SPINE AND TRUNK

The spine is composed of a series of bones, vertebrae, between which nerves pass, connecting the spinal cord to other parts of the body. The main directions of spinal movement are forward and backward bending, side bending and twisting. The spine also permits a degree of longitudinal compression and tension.

The vertebral column consists of five main sections that create four natural front–back curves – the cervical, thoracic, lumbar and sacral curves:
- The cervical spine (seven vertebrae at the neck)
- The thoracic spine (12 vertebrae behind the chest)
- The lumbar spine (five vertebrae that make up the lower back)
- The sacrum (five vertebrae that fuse between the ages of 16 and 30)
- The coccyx (four vertebrae that fuse between the ages of 20 and 30).

The human spine performs several key functions:
- It encases and protects the spinal cord
- Supports the head and enables balance through the weight-bearing column of vertebra and discs
- Provides scaffolding for the muscles, bones and ligaments that attach to it
- Empowers the trunk and limbs to execute a vast array of diverse movements, ranging from those requiring complex shapes changes as in yoga, dancing and other athletic skills
- Acts as a shock absorber to protect the brain while walking, running and performing vigorous weight-bearing activities.

The body is held in its upright stance against the force of gravity in three-dimensional space via the balance of not only these spinal curves, but also the symmetry of the left and right sides. In an ideal upright posture seen from the side, the ankle, knee, hip, shoulder and ear should be in line, and the front and back views should exhibit a bilateral symmetry.

The sacrum provides the platform for most of the spine and is firmly wedged like a keystone between the pelvic bones at the sacro-iliac joints, which in turn balance on the legs at the hip joints. If this platform is disturbed through injury or postural changes, the portion of the spine above it has to compensate, creating a knock-on effect right up to the head.

The vertebral column relies on a variety of soft tissues to support it. Passive support is achieved through non-contractile connective tissue, namely intervertebral discs, ligaments and fascia. The intervertebral discs cushion and separate the vertebrae, ligaments link the vertebrae in a longitudinal direction and fascia provides additional attachments and layers but is thinner and more widespread.

Active support is provided by various muscle groups attaching directly to the spine, pelvis and ribs. These are collectively known as the erector spinae. Beneath this layer are smaller muscles that permit more intricate segmental movements to mediate the more powerful movements of the erectors. Important muscles in terms of both movement and posture are the psoas, which originate from the front of the lumbar spine and attach to the top of each leg. When they are overly taut, as with the erector spinae, these muscles can cause postural deviation and back pain.

Indirect support is also vital to create a coherent and stable upright posture and is provided by cavity pressures in the thorax and abdomen. These are influenced by the health of the lungs and abdominal organs (viscera), as well as by the tone of the thoracic/abdominal muscles, diaphragm and pelvic floor.

COMMON BACK CONDITIONS

Back and neck pain have many forms but the most common are mechanical problems related to the spine's structure and therefore precipitated by certain movements. Modern medical thinking often splits such complaints into categories like muscle, joint and ligament damage, disc damage and sciatica. However, in reality it is often a combination of some or all of these that cause 'mechanical' back pain. There is, nevertheless, also the possibility of 'non-mechanical' back pain. This includes referred pain from internal organs, infection or occasionally even cancer.

Muscles and ligaments are the tissues most commonly damaged. A tear or other injury here is often the external symptom of an underlying imbalance within the skeletal structure, possibly a spinal joint problem. Thoracic pain may additionally be associated with damage to the ribs or respiratory conditions. In the cervical and lumbar regions the smaller 'facet' joints at the rear of the vertebrae are often the culprits, as opposed to the more durable intervertebral discs, although both may be implicated simultaneously.

Disc pain is usually due to a strain or tear in its cartilaginous fibres, called an annulus fibrosus, and tends to be long-lasting and recurrent. Discs can also bulge, usually just to one side, which is known in laymen's terms as a 'slipped disc'. This can result in either local back pain or the radiation of a sharp or burning pain along the sciatic nerve to the leg – a condition known as sciatica, which can be due to arthritic spurs and muscular entrapment. Arms may also be subject to the equivalent of sciatica due to similar causes. A prolapsed disc, when the internal nucleus bursts out of the surrounding cartilage, is the most severe disc injury and usually follows a traumatic incident, such as a bad fall, car accident, or lifting a heavy weight. The prolapse may, however, take years to occur.

Osteoarthritis, also called spondylosis, is a degenerative condition characterized by wear and tear of the cartilage around the joints. In the case of spinal osteoarthritis, it is the erosion of the intervertebral discs, which normally cushion vertical impact. Gradual deterioration of these discs is one of the key reasons we tend to get shorter as we grow old. The symptoms commonly experienced with osteoarthritis are stiffness and severe aches and pains, which alleviate with gentle movement and/or heat. The areas usually worst affected are the lower lumbar spine and the neck.

THERAPIES AND TREATMENTS

The 'medicine' most often prescribed for back problems is simply rest, plus analgesics or anti-inflammatories, although surgery is sometimes advised in extreme cases. Alternative treatment methods include structural therapy, such as osteopathy and remedial massage, acupuncture and yoga therapy.

Stress and tension are major factors in back and neck pain, yet these are often sadly overlooked and frequently underestimated as causes. A lack of exercise and too much time sitting in chairs and/or cars are also significant factors in the Western world; human beings were designed to walk! Walking involves a substantial degree of spinal movement with the joints of the lumbar spine, in particular, playing a key role in locomotion. This makes even the 'simple' task of walking a very different proposition when suffering from acute lower back pain.

Other courses of action you can take are:
- Avoid long periods of sitting in chairs, and at home try to sit in a variety of positions on the floor
- Walk at least 30 minutes every day
- In the summer, walk barefoot or on grass or sand
- Buy shoes that do not cramp the toes and keep heels at a sensible height. High heels create excessive 'swayback' and can be an important variable in managing lower back pain
- Reduce your intake of sugar and acid-forming foods, such as dairy products, meat and refined flour products
- Weight loss, if appropriate, will reduce the strain on the spinal discs, allowing them to absorb more fluid
- Ensuring good hydration of the body may also have dramatic effects.

The vinyasas in this chapter have been specifically chosen to ease any discomfort or pain in the back, and can be combined with a visualization of healing breathing to the site of the problem.

Beginner's Back Vinyasa

A gentle, progressive adaptation of the sun salutation (see pages 52–55), this vinyasa will promote flexibility in the spine. Steps 1–3 are suitable for all levels of ability, while intermediate students can practise the full ten steps. The sequence may be repeated several times on rising in the morning to prepare you for the day ahead. It will help alleviate stiffness in the spine and surrounding muscles, promoting psychosomatic connections. If you experience any pain, rest and breathe in child's pose.

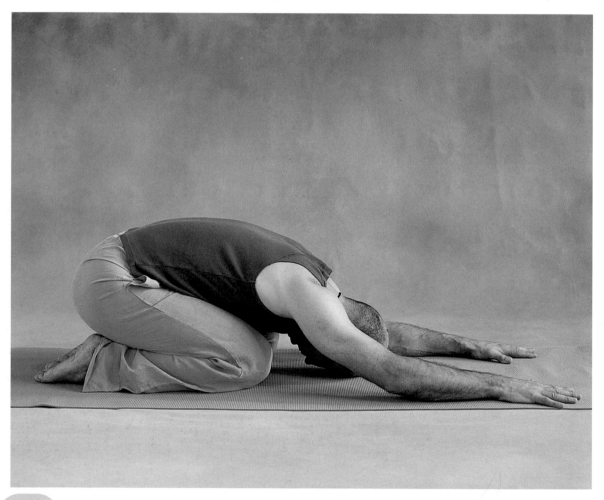

1 Sit on your heels in child's pose (see page 45). Extend your arms out in front of you with the palms flat on the floor to stretch the upper body and lengthen the abdomen. Relax the lower back and abdomen, and practise belly breathing for ten breaths (see page 30).

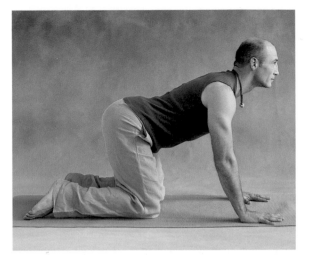
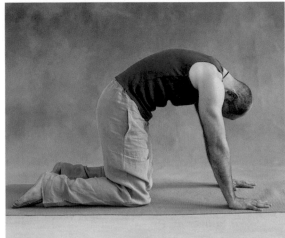

2 On inhale, rise onto all fours to the tabletop position. Place your hands beneath your shoulders and your knees beneath your hips. Press the palms down to the floor. On inhale, dip the spine, stretching the abdomen, chest and throat, and look up. Lift your tailbone as high as you can.

On exhale, curl the spine. Tuck your tailbone under and tuck your chin towards the chest, separating the scapulae (shoulder blades). Squeeze out the breath, engaging the three bandhas (see pages 16–17). Repeat the two movements in synchrony with the breath for 10–20 times until the back is limber and the mind is soft.

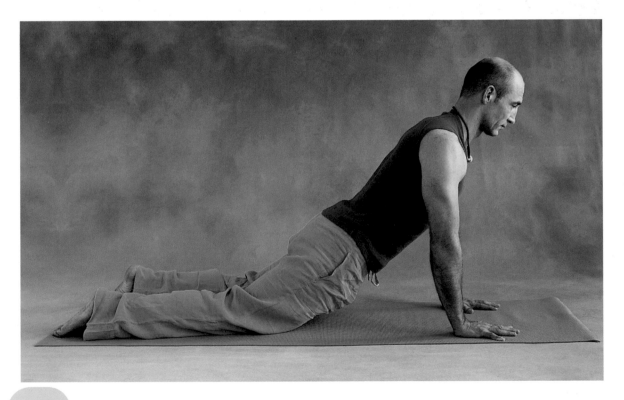

3 Now place the hands further forwards along the yoga mat. As you inhale, draw the chest forwards between the arms in a modified plank pose, lifting upwards and creating a straight line between the knees and the head. Look forwards and monitor

any discomfort in the lower back. On exhale, relax back to the extended child's pose (see step 1) to counterstretch the spine for ten breaths. Repeat steps 1–3 three to five times. This stretch provides relief for severely tight backs.

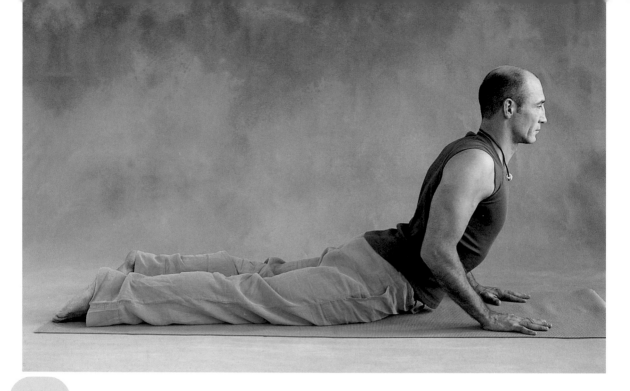

4 Developing from step 3, as long as there is no strain, lower your upper body and draw the chest forwards, bending the elbows into the sides of the waist in a 'baby' cobra posture (bhujangasana).

Articulate the thoracic spine, dipping it between the shoulder blades, broaden the chest and look straight ahead. Monitor any discomfort in your lower back. Hold the position for ten breaths.

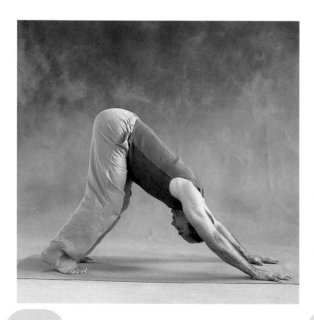

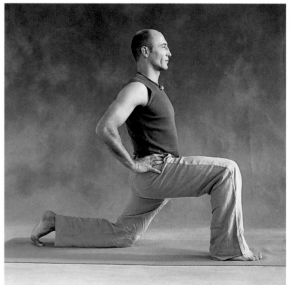

5 From baby cobra, tuck the toes under and, on exhale, lift into the 'puppy', a downward dog pose modified by bending the knees to stretch and lengthen out the spine and 'tune' the hamstrings and lower back (see also page 40). Hold for eight breaths as long as there is no strain.

6 On inhale, step forward with the right foot into a lunge position. Bring your torso to vertical and place your hands on your hips, lifting the front of the armpits. Anchor the tailbone towards the floor, look straight ahead and hold for three breaths.

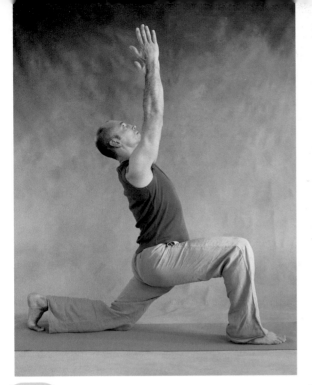

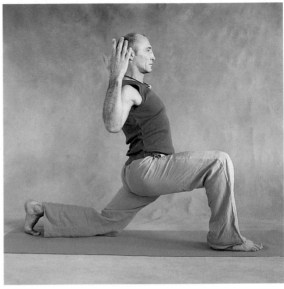

7 On inhale, reach both arms up vertically from the shoulders, drawing in the lower abdomen. Broaden and anchor down the shoulder blades. Turn the palms facing by rotating the biceps. Hold for five breaths.

8 On exhale, draw the elbows to earth, bringing the hands down to ear level. Then, on inhale, extend the arms up again as in step 7. Repeat three times.

Back Vinyasa:
BENEFITS & EFFECTS

- Child's pose helps to flex and lengthen the lower back, particularly good in reducing excessive lordosis (spine curvature, or 'swayback').
- Cat pose limbers the whole spine in flexion and extension, drawing fresh blood towards deep spinal structures and muscles, and mobilizing the neck.
- Plank develops core strength of the thoraco-abdomino-pelvic pressure system and develops upper-body strength.
- Baby cobra lengthens the abdomen, simultaneously easing the spine into extension.
- Lunging promotes hip flexibility and, in combination with arm raises, stretches abdominal muscles and elevates the viscera. (Sluggish abdominal organs can exert strain on the lower back and this sequence helps to strengthen the abdominals.)
- The twisting variation focuses on stretching the psoas muscle and helps to squeeze the intervertebral discs, promoting fresh blood flow in the spinal area. (Because the psoas and abdominals work together, psoas muscles pull the lumbar spine forward; abdominals help to resist this tendency – it is important to balance both sets of muscles.)

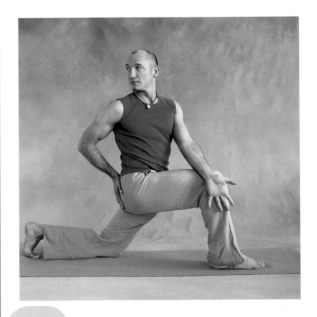

9 On exhale, twist the body to right, placing the back of your left hand outside your right knee, and placing the palm of your right hand on the sacrum. Gently twist to the right and hold for ten breaths, maintaining uddiyana bandha (see page 17). Avoid slumping into the front hip and lower back. Finish by resting back on your heels in child's pose for ten breaths. Then lift the hips into downward puppy and repeat steps 5–9 on the left side before resting in child's pose.

Intermediate Standing Vinyasa

This sequence strengthens the ankles, thighs, calves and spine, facilitating dynamic alignment and improving spinal flexibility. The chair pose, utkatasana, helps track the knees over the parallel feet in a powerful half squat. It is vital to drop anchor with the tailbone and engage the pelvic floor and lower abdomen to protect the lumbar curve, connecting to the 'inner unit' of core support intrinsic to lower back health.

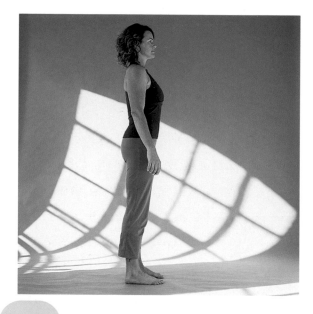

1 Stand in mountain pose, tadasana, with your arms by your sides and your feet parallel. Anchor your big toes and inner heels, and lift your inner ankles.

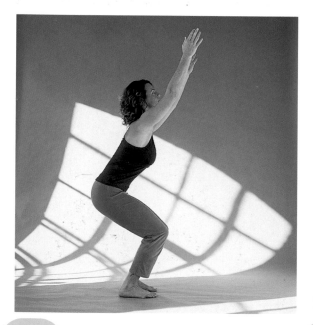

2 On inhale, raise your arms without lifting the shoulders, keeping them forward and parallel, palms facing. Exhale and bend your knees in the chair pose (utkatasana), aiming to draw the thighs parallel to the floor. The torso will lean slightly forward over the thighs. Hold for five to ten breaths.

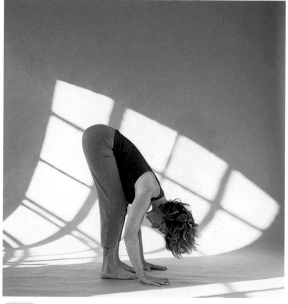

3 On exhale, straighten your legs a little and lower your arms to the floor to sweep into a forward bend. If necessary, bend your knees and place your palms flat on the floor. Release the cervical spine and press your belly on your thighs. Hold for five to ten breaths and on inhale return to mountain pose.

Archetypal Spiral Twist

This strong, robust movement for more advanced students is designed to follow a long, gravitational pathway through the spine. Synchronized with the breath, the ascending and descending diagonal movements are liberating and empowering. Avoid this exercise, however, if you suffer from back pain.

Archetypal Spiral:
BENEFITS & EFFECTS

- With its sidebend and rotation movements, this sequence grooms the archetypal spiral around which the human physique is designed.
- The action of 'throwing a spear' demands an initial rotation of the spine away from the target and a slight shifting of body weight to the rear, followed by a rotation towards the target and slight shifting of weight forwards – enhancing proprioceptive ability of the body to balance itself.
- This pose alternately stretches and compresses adjacent layers of the abdominal wall and inter-vertebral spinal discs (as both structures possess diagonally orientated fibres).
- The sequence creates an alternating deep spiral stretch and compression of the abdominal contents, promoting free movement of the viscera and revitalizing their circulation.

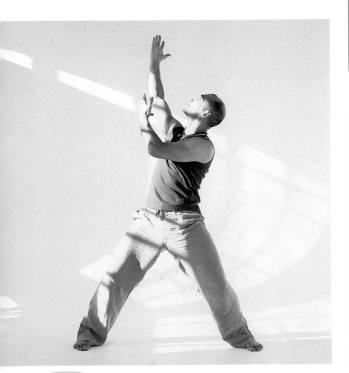

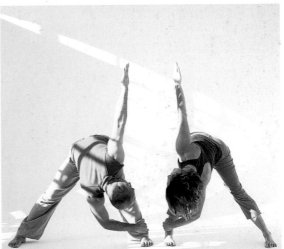

1 Stand facing forwards with your legs wide apart and arms by your sides. On inhale, twist to the top right diagonal, reaching both arms upwards, as if you are about to throw a spear. Look up to the hands.

2 On exhale, rotate your upper body and arms down through the diagonal plane, ending with the right hand outside your left shin, followed by the left hand reaching back to the sky. Look to the side of the left foot and bend your knees, if necessary. Repeat the sequence five times, and then change sides.

Intermediate Side Flank
Vinyasa

In the following dynamic sequence a symmetrical bend, padottanasana, combines with an asymmetrical side flank, parsvakonasana, which extends the spine, tones the hips and opens up the upper lung. Both lengthen the spine and strengthen the back. Using the hands for support improves safety and acts as a counterpose. If you have lower back problems, bend the knees in the forward bend (step 2) and modify the sequence.

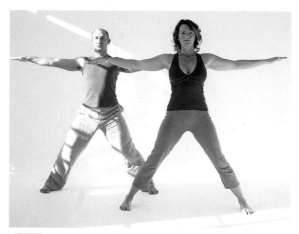

1 Stand with legs approximately 1 m (3 ft) wide apart and your inner feet parallel to each other with your arms by your sides. On inhale, extend your arms straight out to the sides, stretching your fingertips and look forwards. Breathe deeply for three breaths.

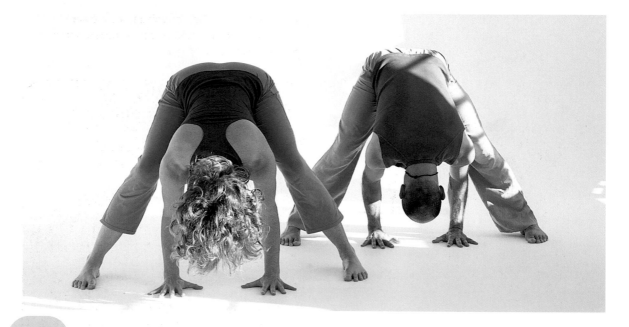

2 On exhale, bend your knees directly over your toes. Hinge forwards from the front hips and place the hands on the floor between the feet. Bend the knees as much as necessary to reduce strain in the back. Release the neck, allowing the head to drop comfortably down between the shoulders. Stretch the toes and fingers from their roots. This is called prasarita padottanasana. Hold for ten breaths.

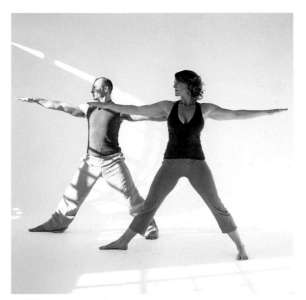

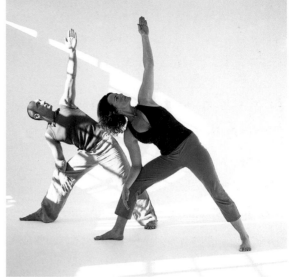

3 On inhale, return to standing. Lift and lengthen your front torso and stretch your arms out to the sides as in step 1. Turn your left hip and foot inwards, and turn your right foot and hip outwards about 90 degrees on exhale. Gaze to the right so you are looking over your right foot and outstretched right arm.

4 On inhale, lift the chest and anchor the tailbone. Then, on exhale tilt the upper body to the right without straining. Bending your right leg slightly, place the right elbow on the right thigh and stretch the left arm up to the sky. Bend the knee as much as necessary to minimize strain on the lower back. Look up at your left arm and hold for five to eight breaths, depending on ability. Repeat steps 3 and 4 several times before returning to centre and repeating on the left side. Imagine you are moving between two panes of glass.

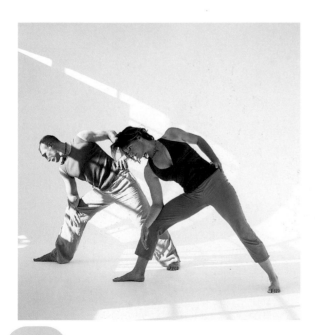

5 Now look down to your right foot and, to stabilize, bring your left arm to rest on your left hip. Loosen the neck. On inhale, return to step 1 and repeat the whole sequence for the left side of the body.

Side Angle and Forward Bends:
BENEFITS & EFFECTS

- Padottanasana allows the lower back to be stretched gently using gravity, with minimal stress on the hamstrings.
- In the forward bend, the facet joints and capsules of the spine are subjected to a traction (decompressive) force.
- The bend strengthens and stretches the inner and back legs and the spine.
- The side movement, parsvakonasana (step 4), stretches one side of the body to create freedom of both external musculature and internal organs. Performed bilaterally, it helps to redress asymmetry in the body, in particular the lateral muscles of the torso and spine.
- The abdominal organs are toned, the brain is calmed and mild backache may be relieved.

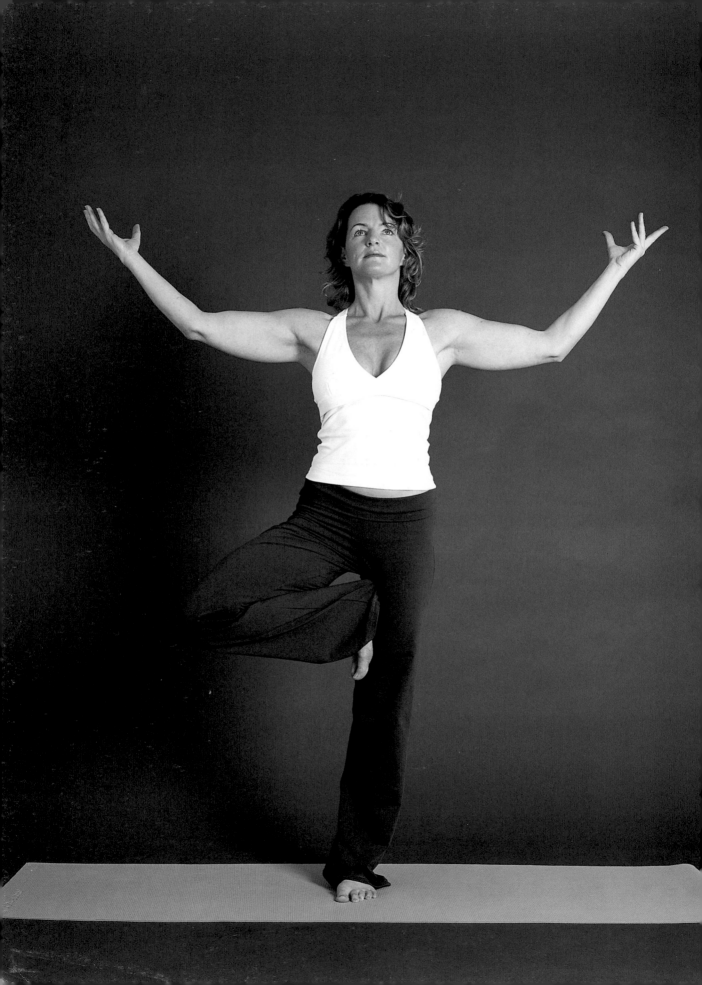

the lymphatic and immune systems: building up resistance

One of the main principles of yoga therapy is cultivating the ability to let go of attachment to objects, events, people, mental constructs and emotions. This is a brave undertaking, yet at the same time holds the key to true 'liberation in life' (jivanmukti). A huge amount of energy is required to keep repressed material outside awareness (that is, to hide it in the unconscious). But if we can let go of repressed material, energy for healing and vitality is released. Restrictive emotions and anxieties can lead to 'dis-ease', our body not in harmony, and ultimately chronic illness. Spiritual traditions suggest that we open our eyes to a deeper seeing by creating a healing space with what is called 'sankalpa', a trusting acceptance of what is, while letting go of barriers.

Loneliness and lack of support is also considered a factor in weakening health, and positive suggestion and emotional support strengthen immune responses. We have all experienced the comfort that stroking an animal brings, and the safe touch of another. A healing environment therefore needs to provide emotional care, and in an integrated yoga practice, emotions are observed as closely as the physical body: the practice offers a mirror for self-reflection.

THE IMMUNE SYSTEM

The system is the body's watchdog that never sleeps, continually preventing foreign substances from entering the body and attacking those inside with an assortment of white blood cells, each with a specific role. It is a highly complex secret army of white blood cells, bone marrow, antibodies, cytokines (substances produced by cells of the immune system that can affect the system's response to attack) and the thymus gland (which produces T-cells). A strong immune function identifies 'nonself' and 'self' cells and fights off 'nonself' foreign bodies. However, when the body's fighter cells are weakened due to too much stress in the system (oversecretions of adrenaline and cortisol, and too much sympathetic 'excitory' nervous activity), the immune function becomes sluggish against bacteria, viruses, cancer cells and fungi. In such cases, autoimmune disease can occur.

A strong immune system is boosted by good sattwic, a natural and unpolluted diet, fresh air, positive pursuits and relaxation, low stress and minimal stimulants. It is no coincidence that when we feel low or weak, and are susceptible to disease, we say, 'I'm not feeling myself today.' Psychically, getting rid of what we do not need – mental, emotional or physical baggage – will free and boost immunity, enhancing zest for life.

THE LYMPHATIC SYSTEM

The lymphatic system is important to the body's defense mechanisms because it helps filter out organisms that cause disease. It also produces white blood cells, generates antibodies, distributes fluids and nutrients and drains excess fluid and protein to avoid tissue swelling.

The lymphatic system begins developing in the fifth week of intrauterine life: lymph, lymphatic vessels and lymphoid tissue (specialized reticular tissue containing large numbers of lymphocytes), in such organs as the thymus gland, spleen, lymph nodes and tonsils.

The lymph vessels begin as capillaries which drain the interstitial fluid between cells, joining like a river to become larger and larger vessels, which ultimately drain into the thoracic duct or the right lymphatic duct on either side of the spine. The lymphatic system is therefore a one-way system, which is essential for removing waste from cells. Because of the one-way system, lymphatic vessels have more valves and also thicker walls. Lymph enters the systemic circulation through the subclavian veins – veins under the collarbones. It is a milky fluid that contains lymphocytes (white blood cells), along with proteins and fats.

Lymph nodes are oval structures located along lymphatic vessels. They filter incoming lymph, which then continues past the node to the larger vessels. The nodes are strategically located in such areas as the armpit and groin, thereby acting to prevent the spread of infection to more vital areas of the body. Lymph nodes filter and process lymph via a process called phagocytosis, the ingestion of foreign material, and through T-cells and B-cells, which produce antibodies.

The spleen produces antibody-producing plasma cells, carries out phagocytosis on bacteria and damaged red blood cells, and stores and releases blood.

The thymus gland produces T-lymphocytes, from stem cells in the embryonic bone marrow, and distributes them to all the lymphatic organs. The thymus confers what is known as 'immunological competence' on the T-cells, enabling them to differentiate into a variety of cells with specific immune functions.

The tonsils and the skin are the body's front line of defence, the sentries guarding the gate. They produce lymphocytes and antibodies.

Bone marrow also produces lymphocytes, and so can also be considered as part of the immune system.

RESISTANCE TO DISEASE

The body resists disease using two different mechanisms: non-specific immunity and specific immunity. Non-specific relates to the mechanical workings of the body that have a protective effect. These include the skin, mucous membranes, mucous, saliva, cilia (small hairs), lachrymal apparatus, epiglottis and urine flow. These physical methods are complemented by chemical substances that also help to fight infection, such as the acidity of the skin and gastric juice, unsaturated fatty acids in sebum and lysozyme in fluids such as sweat, tears and saliva.

Resistance to specific diseases, or immunity, develops throughout life, but particularly during faetal life and childhood, by the production of specific lymphocytes and antibodies (different forms of white blood cells) against a specific antigen (a substance that stimulates the production of an antibody). The efficiency of the immune system tends to decline with old age. In addition, the destruction of antigens by T-cells is known as cellular immunity and the destruction of antigens by B-cells is called humoral immunity. This later mechanism, whereby antigens are 'remembered' by their respective antibody, is the physiological basis for immunization - the model upon which we base our vaccination methods. T-cells are produced in the thymus gland and lymph nodes, whereas B-cells may be processed in bone marrow, fetal liver and spleen, and lymphoid tissue of the gut. They develop into antibody-producing plasma cells. The body actually produces thousands of B- and T-cells, each one capable of responding to a specific antigen.

COMMON IMMUNE DISORDERS

T-cells – the body's fighter cells produced by the thymus gland – flood the system in states of intense emotion, including happiness and sadness. This implies that exploring and expressing emotions strengthens and boosts the immune system, and can affect heart, nervous, immune and respiratory functions.

In a healthy body the tissues of the body are recognized by T- and B-cells as being part of the body. This state, known as immunological tolerance, can break down and lead to a variety of disorders called auto-immune diseases, in which the body's own tissue antigens are recognized as foreign by the immune system. Antibodies are produced, which then attack these specific tissues.

So-called auto-immune diseases include rheumatoid arthritis, multiple sclerosis, hyperthyroidism, glomerular nephritis (kidney disease) and Addison's disease. The reason for this phenomena has not been fully explained by medical research, although the structures involved may offer a clue as to the underlying cause; namely, the tissues of the central nervous system, the endocrine system and the kidney. These tissues are all involved in dealing with the stress response and it is likely that prolonged exposure to stress may be the trigger to what amounts to an 'immune system breakdown'. Along with stress, triggers can be from viral infections, a hormonal imbalance or environmental toxins.

In addition to the ailments below, general complaints can be evidence of a weakened immune system and responses of the body to infection include inflammation and fever. Allergies can be the result of a generally sluggish or poor-functioning immune system. Cancer and depression can be side-effects of an under-supported immune system, and recurrent infections, such as colds, viruses and urinary tract infections, can also occur with a weakened immune system.

Chronic fatigue syndrome is a disorder characterized by extreme physical and mental fatigue. Symptoms can include muscle and joint aches, swollen glands due to recurrent infections, depression and digestive disorders.

AIDS, Acquired Immune-Deficiency Syndrome, develops following an infection with the Human Immunodeficiency Virus (HIV), which is usually transmitted sexually or by contaminated blood or needles. The virus destroys the T-lymphocytes, which combat infection, so that the immune system becomes progressively weakened.

THERAPIES AND TREATMENTS

Conventional drugs are administered to boost the production of white blood cells and to fight off invaders. In addition to the asanas in this chapter, sun salutations (see pages 52–55) will help to boost your immune system by increasing pranic energy and balancing nervous and endocrine function.

Other lifestyle recommendations that may improve the immune system and overall health are:
- Adequate and regular sleep
- Eating a nutritionally sound diet rich in antioxidants (found in dark orange, yellow, red and green vegetables) and immune-enhancing probiotic yogurt, green tea and garlic
- Reducing intake of coffee, alcohol, tobacco, saturated fats and refined sugar
- Taking a fruit or a fast day once a week or month to clear the body of accumulated toxins
- Exercise and such treatements as massage and dry-skin brushing to help the body eliminate toxins
- Relaxing the mind with yoga nidra (see page 123) and engaging in positive thinking.

Sankalpa and Mantras

A Sanskrit word meaning 'resolve' or 'resolution', sankalpa is a short statement formed to open a pathway of healing by planting a positive seed of change into the subconscious mind through thought power. A potent force in healing, sankalpa conjures enormous willpower and endurance and is especially useful in chronic diseases, such as cancer, to heal and give courage.

'Manas' means to think, and 'tra' to protect or free oneself. A repeated sound, word or phrase, mantras are employed as a way of generating positive, creative intention, transcending limiting and restrictive thought patterns. Mantras are generally practised following pranayama and relaxation. The symbol and sound 'Om' is known as the first sound, 'the sound birth of the cosmic mind'. Seen as a parallel to 'Amen' and 'Shalom', it is considered to be the first utterance from which creation manifests. Om is associated with the higher chakras of ajna, the 'third eye', and sahasrara (see also pages 14–15 and 122).

The Tree Pose (Vrksasana)

The tree pose strengthens the legs, ankles and spine. It stretches the inner thighs, improves a sense of balance, relieves sciatica and helps flat feet. With its arm-raising action, this sequence revitalizes the body and opens the mind to positive energy.

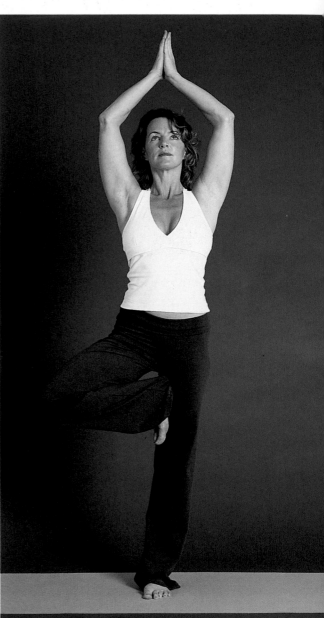

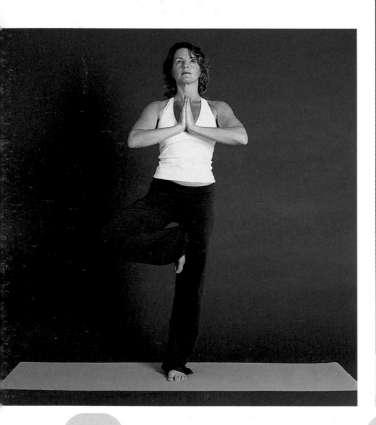

1 Stand in the mountain pose, tadasana (see page 52). Shift your weight onto the left foot, grounding all corners of the foot, but lifting the inner arch. Bend your right knee and draw your right foot up, placing it against the inner left thigh, toes pointing towards the floor. Wing open your right hip and anchor your tailbone towards earth. Place your hands in the prayer position, namaste, with palms pressed together and the elbows out to the sides. Look ahead and breathe for five to ten breaths.

2 On inhalation, raise your hands, still pressed together, above your head. Lift your sternum and lengthen through both sides of your trunk. Root the standing foot deeply.

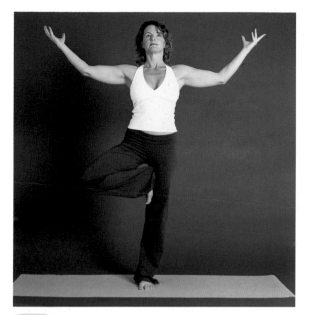

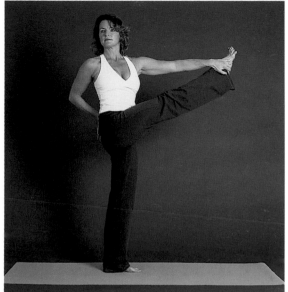

3 Now branch open your arms, with the palms to the sky and fingers outstretched. Hold for five to ten breaths. Return to mountain pose on exhalation and repeat the sequence standing on the right leg. Ground from the pelvis through the legs to earth. Ascend from the lumbar upwards through the spine.

Advanced: From the tree pose in step 1, raise the right leg straight in front and, if stable, hold the outside edge of your right foot with your left hand and fully extend the leg. Place your right hand on your lower back for support. Hold for five to ten breaths. Return to mountain pose and repeat sequence on the other side.

Lord of the Dance (Natarajasana)

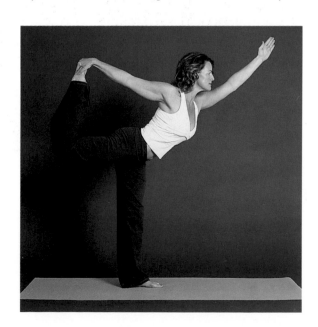

This posture develops balance and strengthens the legs. Standing postures help give the body immune-boosting resistance and strength.

1 Stand in mountain pose, tadasana. Standing strong on your left foot, on inhalation grasp your right foot with your right hand and lift it behind you. Stretch your left hand to vertical above your head.

2 Breathing steadily, slowly lift your right foot up and away from your body. Extend the right leg behind you, parallel to the floor, arching your spine as you lift. Simultaneously stretch your left arm out straight in front of you. Breathe for ten breaths, then release back to standing. Repeat with the arms and legs reversed.

Peacock Tail (Pincha-mayurasana)

An advanced, challenging version of the peacock (see pages 79–80), this pose develops upper-body and core strength, enabling you to distribute the backbend throughout the spinal stem to re-energize and rebalance. Caution: this is only for experienced yoga pupils. It should not be attempted unless you are fully fit and have mastered the peacock pose.

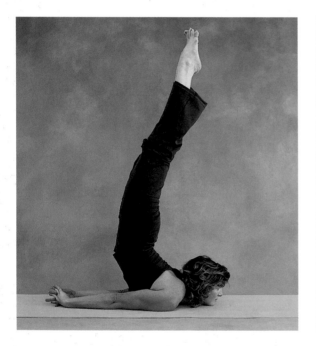

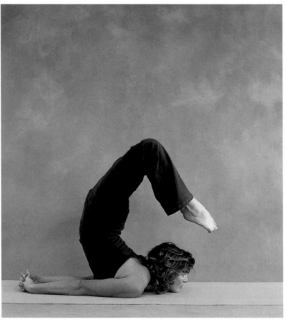

1 Lie face down on your mat, placing the clasped hands together underneath your pubic bone. Broaden your shoulders and open your chest.

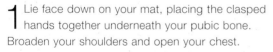

2 Press the legs together and lift the straight legs off the floor, holding the locust pose, salabhasana. If you can, flip your legs up one at a time, harnessing uddiyana bandha, to stretch the legs skywards. Squeeze the legs together and extend through the soles of your feet. Hold for five to ten breaths, if possible. To release, come back down, one leg at a time, and counterpose in child's pose, balasara (see page 45), or lower both legs simultaneously (via step 3) to lie on your belly.

Variation: Carefully bend your knees and drop your feet towards your head. Hold for five to ten breaths, then slowly lift your legs to vertical before releasing the pose as in step 2. Arch your thoracic spine powerfully.

Eagle Pose (Garudasana)

The eagle pose encourages strength, endurance and concentration, which can help stabilize you mentally and physically. Do not practise if you have knee injuries – instead, just bend the knees.

1 Stand in mountain pose, tadasana. Bend your knees slightly, lift your right foot up and, balancing on your left leg, cross your right thigh over the left. Hook the top of the foot behind the lower left calf and squat deep.

2 Stretch your arms out straight in front of you, and cross the right arm over the left at the elbows. Raise the forearms to vertical. (The palms of the hands should face each other.) Press the palms together and lift the elbows higher, stretching the fingers skywards. Draw your shoulder blades down your back.

3 Breathe for eight breaths, then unravel the legs and arms, and stand in mountain pose again. Repeat on the other side.

Inversions and Balances: BENEFITS & EFFECTS

- Inversions revive and restore the whole system, literally taking the weight off your legs and bathing the heart and brain in healthy blood flow.
- Inversions send oxygen to the brain and reverse gravity, which leads to clearer thinking, improved circulation, and relieves sluggishness in the organs.
- Balances are centring, tethering you to the present moment, and encouraging clarity and awareness of what is. Driving the feet into the earth, yet springing up and spiralling through the spine, one's inner connection and creative source is enhanced.
- They help to improve the drainage of the lymphatic vessels, thereby assisting the function of the overall immune system.

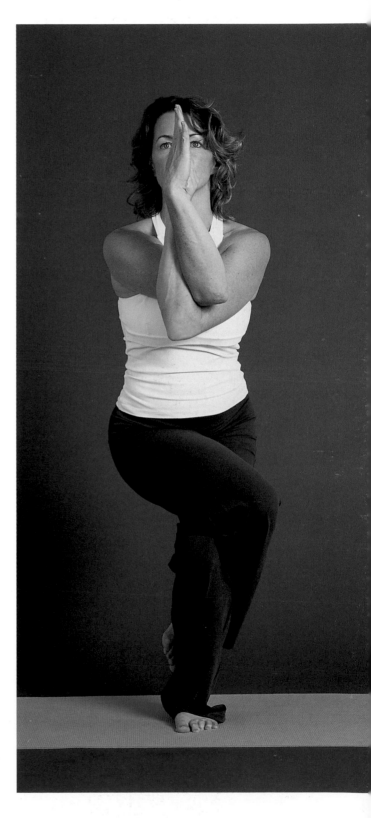

Supported Fish Pose

If you are suffering from an immune-deficiency illness or are run-down, resting in poses for three-to-five-minute holds, supported by cushions, bolsters and a wall, will engender healing. According to ancient texts, the fish pose is meant to be the 'destroyer of all diseases'.

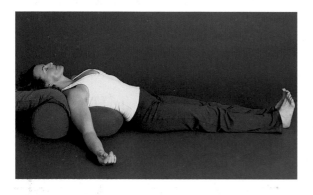

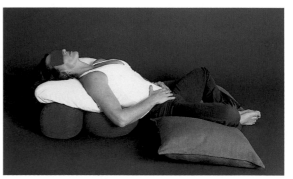

Option one: Lie on your back on the floor and place a bolster or cushion under the upper back in order to keep the chest elevated and the head and neck supported. Align the body carefully as if you are practising the full fish posture (see page 76), but become a resting fish!

Option two: You can achieve more relaxed support by cushioning beneath the thighs in butterfly pose (supta baddha konasana, see page 71). Place a cushion under your thighs to protect the knees, keeping your hips on the floor. Keep the soles of your feet together and the palms resting on your lower abdomen.

Supported Downward Dog

Downward dog rests the heart and bathes the brain with fresh blood. Resting the brow on a bolster can further soothe the brain and the brow. Experiment with the height of the cushion or bolster so the neck is not cramped. Rest up to three minutes.

Place a bolster or cushion on the floor. Practise downward dog (see page 40) and rest the hairline of the head on the bolster. Lengthen through the arms and spine for one minute. Counterpose in child's pose (see page 45) with the brow resting on the bolster.

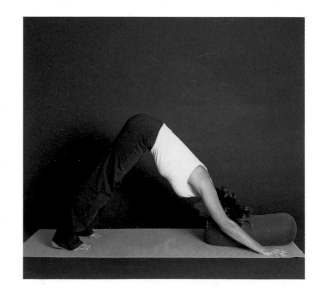

Supported Relaxation

Resting the body in passive relaxation with the legs raised gives time for bodily systems to come back into equilibrium. This pose is ideal for recuperation or meditation.

Place a straight-back chair at one end of your mat and a broad, flat, padded cushion in front of it. Lie down, face up, with your whole torso on the cushion and your head slightly lower on the mat. Place the calves on the seat of the chair so that the legs form a right angle and the feet are flat against the chair back. Now rest your hands on the lower abdomen, palms down. Breathe deeply for as long as is comfortable.

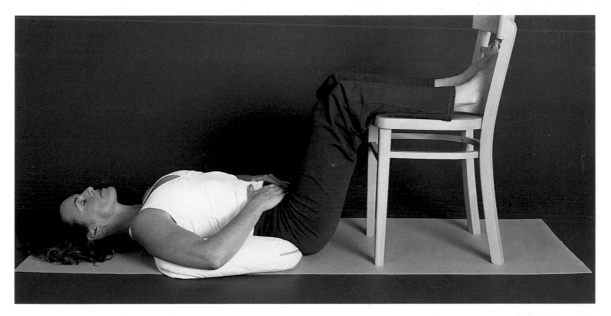

Supported Shoulderstand

The shoulderstand helps the lymph/immune system in many ways. It soothes the nervous system, enhances blood circulation and brings balance to other systems of the body.

Begin in the rest pose, above, but with your shoulders on the cushion and your head carefully resting lower than your shoulders. Holding the chair legs for support with straight arms, slide your feet to the front of the chair seat and lift the hips and back. Raise the knees towards the ceiling; keep the back of the neck relaxed.

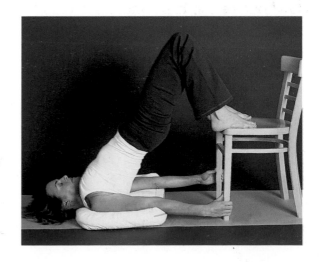

Energy-charging Mudra (Shivalingam)

In this gesture we form a pestle and mortar with the hands, symbolizing the lingum (phallus) of Shiva, the first yogi. Negative patterns that hold us back are placed mentally in the pestle, and the grinding action dispels these thought constructs into a fine dust, which is then blown away into 'ka' (space).

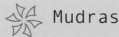

Mudras

Healing requires positive energy and tremendous focus, and rituals and symbolic gestures give a framework to strengthen the mind, just as asanas provide a framework to strengthen the body. Mudras are gestures, seals or symbols, usually with the hands, which engender a certain attitude in the mind and link nerve pathways, too. Our bodily gestures affect our mind deeply and subtle gestures can have far-reaching effects. Mudras create an energy field that helps in healing; they are used alongside breathing exercises (pranayamas), affirmations or mantras, or to enhance meditation and visualization. They can be practised for 10 to 45 minutes and result in an attuned mental attitude.

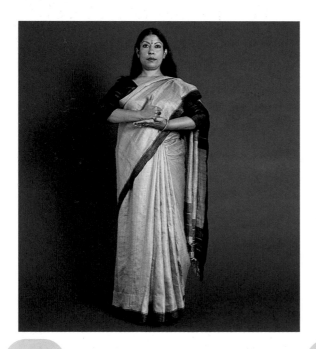

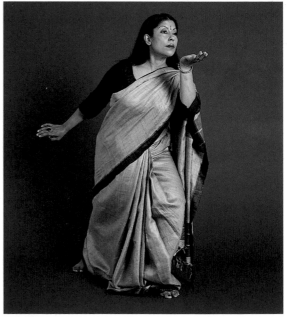

1 Sit comfortably with a straight spine or stand firmly in mountain pose (tadasana). Form your right hand into a fist with the thumb pointing up, like a pestle, and shape your left hand like a shallow bowl or mortar, the fingers close together. Place your right hand on top of your left and put both hands in front of your abdomen.

2 Breathing consciously, mentally place any negative thoughts into the bowl of your left hand. Imagine you are grinding these destructive patterns into a fine dust, circling and pressing the right hand into the left hand palm. Then raise the left hand and gently blow away the dust.

Lotus Flower Mudra

This mudra forms the shape of a lotus flower. Visualize an open-petalled flower which floats on the water, and then sinks its roots deep into the mud and opening its petals to the sky. Create a sankalpa (positive affirmation), such as: 'From that deep ground I'll spring higher.'

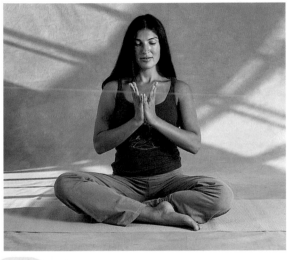

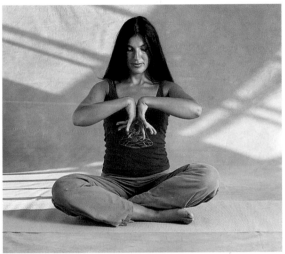

1 Seated comfortably with both sitting bones anchored, hold your hands in front of your heart in prayer position, namaste. Keep the heels of the hands touching to form a bowl and touch the little fingers and the outer edges of the thumbs together. Open out the fingers. Breathing mindfully, repeat your sankalpa.

2 Now close your fingers into a tight bud, joining the backs of the hands and letting the fingers hang down towards the earth. Feel how your fingers are like the plant's deep roots. Repeat several times.

Eagle Wings Mudra (Garuda)

A protecting and strengthening gesture, the eagle wings mudra boosts the circulation and supports the internal organs of the body.

Cross your left hand over your right hand at the wrist and point your fingers upwards. Bring to chest level with the palms facing the body. Now interlock your thumbs and spread out the fingers to form the wings.

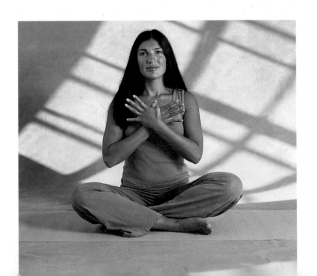

Jnana Mudra

This is one of the classic mudras, used in Hatha yoga meditation and pranayamas; it is also known as 'gyana' mudra. The gesture is said to bestow intelligence and wisdom, purify the mind, cure mental ailments, give a feeling of joy and dislodge addictive habits.

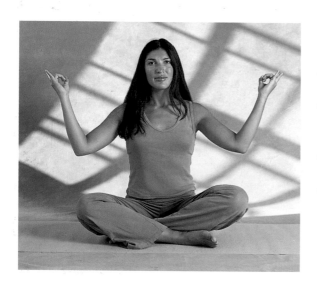

This can be practised in any meditative position, but for energy and vitality, sit in sukhasana with the legs crossed and the feet directly below the knees. Join the tip of the forefinger to the thumb of each hand, as if holding onto a tiny grain of rice, creating a circle with the fingers. Extend out the other three fingers, which signify the three gunas (rajas, sattwa and tamas, see pages 10–11). The index finger signifies the ego, the one which points, blames and identifies. The ego is melted into its source, signified by the thumb, cosmic awareness. Hold for 20 breaths.

Empty Cup Mudra (Bhairava)

The gesture of cupping the void facilitates 'ananta' – spaciousness in the mind. The hands represent ida and pingala nadis (the moon and sun channels) – see page 12. Placing the left on top represents yin – lunar or feminine energy; the reverse indicates yang – solar or masuline energy.

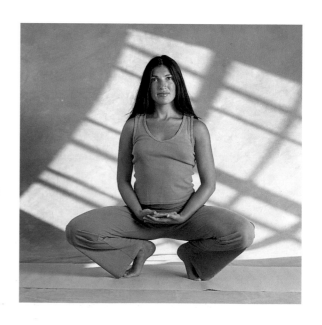

Assume a comfortable meditation posture with the head and spine straight. Place the hands in a cup, so that the palms of both hands are facing up in the lap. Relax the whole body.

Sanmukhi Mudra

This 'sanguine-face' gesture redirects awareness to the self within by closing the seven doors of outer perception – the two eyes, ears and nostrils, and the mouth. By sealing all the sense portals to the outer world, introspection and self-exploration is encouraged. Do not practise if you suffer from depression.

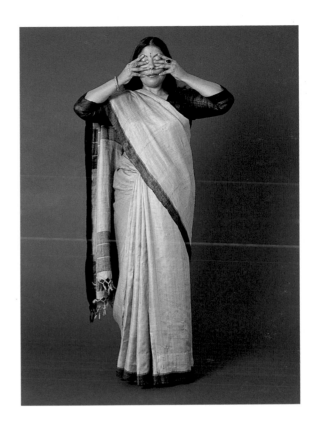

Seated or standing, raise the hands in front of the face with the elbows pointing outwards. Place the index fingers just beneath the eyebrows, the middle fingers gently to press down the eyelids, the ring fingers to press the corners of the nostrils and the little fingers on the corners of the mouth. finally close the lboes of the ears with the thumbs. Rest in this position for one to two minutes, breathing calmly.

Lion Pose

The lion, simhasana, rejuvenates facial muscles and stretches the tongue. A cleansing asana rather than a mudra, it stimulates the sense organs and boosts self-expression.

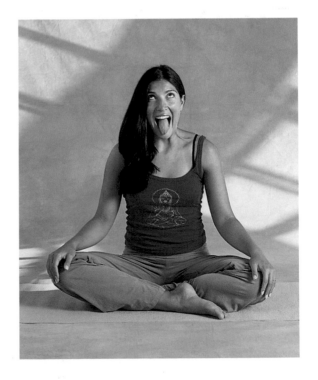

Sit in a comfortable pose and place your hands on your knees. Keeping the mouth closed, breathe slowly and deeply through the nose. At the end of inhalation open the mouth and stretch the tongue out as far as possible towards the chin. While slowly exhaling, produce a clear, steady 'Aaah' sound from the throat, draining the lungs. At the end of exhalation, gaze at your 'third eye', adopting the brow gaze, shambhavi, mudra (see also page 122), and relax the whole body.

Ujjayi Pranayama

Important in health management for its ability to soothe the nerves and strengthen the heart, ujjayi breathing is also said to release the psychic knot in the heart (called vishnu granthi). This has the effect of freeing the emotions from the stranglehold of personal obsession towards the transcendental plane (from 'manas', lower mind, to 'buddhi', higher mind).

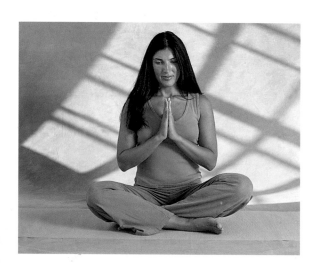

Sit in a comfortable position, such as sukhasana, with the hands in the namaste prayer position, as here. Breathe slowly and smoothly into the thorax by harnessing uddiyana bandha (see page 17), sealing the lower abdominal wall towards the spine. Gently contract mula bandha and jalandhara at the throat (see pages 16–17). This has the effect of siphoning the breath, extracting the 'soul of the air' and stretching the breath, unravelling the thought waves (vrittis) carried in it. In this way the mind is quietened as the breath becomes uncoloured and anxiety is eased. Listen to the sibilant sound produced. Contraction of the glottis is held throughout, and the breath is expanded and stretched into the side ribs, smoothly and consciously. Continue breathing for 20 breaths.

Bee Breath (Bhramari)

The heart chakra is called the centre of the 'unstruck sound', and this nada yoga (sound integration) is a vibrational meditation on the heart, inducing mental and emotional relaxation. A yogic tranquillizer to allay anxiety, the 'bee breath' strengthens the psychic body, acting on the limbic-hypothalamic-pituitary-autonomic axis.

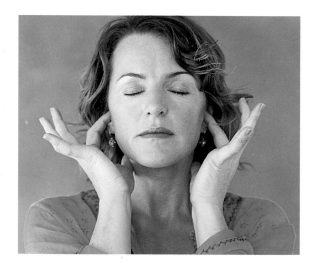

Sit in a comfortable position. Place the index fingers in the lobes of the ears and close the eyes. Now breathe in, smoothly and deeply. Gently hum the outbreath, listening to the inner sound. Repeat without strain. Practise for two to three minutes, two to three times a day, to overcome fear and anxiety.

Nadi Shodana

This pranayama is a harmonizing prelude to meditation and can be used to balance the cardio-respiratory systems and soothe the nervous system. It aims to replicate the state of deep sleep and rapid eye movement (REM), when the brain rests and is replenished, the heart rate slows down and the heart's natural rhythm is restored – which is one beat contraction followed by two beats relaxation, throughout the whole of life. The nadi shodana technique follows this natural rhythm, so here we inhale for a count of one beat and exhale for a count of two beats. Throughout inhalation the heart speeds up; during exhalation the heart slows down, inducing relaxation and health. In addition, channelling breath through alternate nostrils is said to balance the left and right sides of the brain, inducing natural calm.

1 Sitting with a straight spine (which will help improve diaphragmatic descent), press the index and middle fingers of the right hand into the brow centre.

2 Close the right nostril with the thumb of the right hand. The left hand rests upturned on the lap or the left knee. To begin, count your inhales and exhales 1:1. When your breathing is steady and comfortable, vary the count to 1:2. Breathe ten complete breaths in and out through the left nostril. This induces relaxation and internal absorption, activating the parasympathetic limb of the nervous system (ida nadi, lunar energy).

3 Now close the left nostril using the ring finger of the right hand: establish 1:1 inhales and exhales through the right nostril then breathe 1:2 for ten breaths. This activates the flow of pranic energy corresponding with the sympathetic nervous system, externalizing awareness (pingala nadi, solar energy). Now repeat alternating sides for three to four cycles of ten breaths each.

4 Finish by breathing deeply and smoothly through both nostrils. Direct attention to the breath pathways in a triangular pattern, the two incoming streams of air flowing in through left and right nostrils as its two sides, converge at the eyebrow centre, bhrumadhya, and exhaling out again.

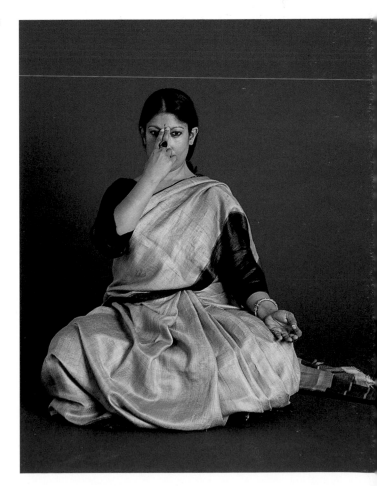

Eyebrow Gaze

This gaze, shambhavi mudra, is good for stress relief, calming the nervous system, stimulating a deeper 'seeing' and balancing left and right.

Gaze inwards and upwards to the eyebrow centre – the 'third eye' – observing your breathing. Focus the eyes to the centre without moving the head. You should see a v-shaped image, which is the two curved eyebrows. Hold the gaze for a total count of 20 breaths. Once you have mastered the eye movement, coordinate it with breathing in slowly as the eyes are raised and breathing out slowly as the gaze is lowered.

Tratak

This eye-cleansing, a kriya from traditional shatkarmas (washings), is also a candle meditation. It promotes ekakrata – one-pointedness and clarity.

Sit in a comfortable position about 1 m (3 ft) in front of a lighted candle. Without closing the eyes, gaze as long as possible at the flame until tears come to the eyes. Close the eyes and visualize the candle flame clearly in the mind's eye for about two minutes. Finally, rub the palms together to warm them and palm the eyes (press them to the eye sockets) several times.

Cancer Visualization

This practice should ideally be given directly from a teacher, but you can ask a friend to read it out to you as you rest in the corpse pose. Before you begin, remove any external stimuli from the room. The act of hearing, listening and feeling are the only requirements. As you become calm, listen to your breathing, and as you breathe out, mentally remind yourself to 'relax'.

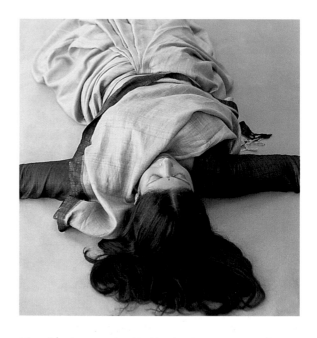

Lie face-up on the floor in the corpse pose, savasna, with your eyes closed, arms by your side and your toes falling outwards. Now stretch your arms out directly to your sides with the palms upwards, so your body is in a 't' formation, an archetypal gesture of surrender. Breathe deeply and allow yourself to rest quietly in the moment with the mind settled.

Visualize the cancer shrinking in size, overcome by a massive surge of white blood cells which slowly and certainly flood the cancer out and bolster the immune response. making your body stronger and healthier with each breath. Visualize your body completely clear of negativity and disease. Feel open and supported as you breathe with ease.

Yoga Nidra

The Unspoken Mantra (Ajapa)

Often referred to as 'psychic sleep', yoga nidra is a healing practice of guided relaxation wherein the parasympathetic nervous system is fully functioning and sympathetic nervous activity is switched off. A bridge is made between the conscious, subconscious and unconscious minds, which guides the practitioner towards the root of their thought patterns where samskaras (habitual tendencies) are recognized and dismantled.

Lie in the supine pose. Concentrate on belly breathing deeply and fully (see page 30). Working your way up the left side of your body and then the right, draw attention to each body part and concentrate on relaxing it, from the toes to the head and finishing with the sense organs – the ears, eyes, nose, mouth and tongue. Naming the body parts allows the brain to be 'stroked' along a pathway that induces deep relaxation. Detach your mind and lie peacefully for ten minutes.

This breathing observation is a meditation practice that charts the pathway of the breath between the navel and the throat, fixing the concentration on the sibilant, whispering sound of the breath and its journey through the spine. Ujjayi means 'to stretch', and the ujjaya breathing employed (see page 17) is a deep, slow, rich, diaphragmatic breathing centred in the thorax. It produces a gentle 'hush' sound due to a subtle contraction of the glottis (the back of the throat). Do not strain while you are breathing.

The ascent and descent of the ujjayi breath between navel and throat is combined with the mantra 'So Ham' in a practice called ajapa japa, which is translated as 'constant awareness' or 'constant remembering'. Ajapa mantra is the unspoken sound of your own breath. Listening to the sound your breath makes draws us closer to our self, our own silence.

To begin, lie in the corpse pose (see opposite). Practise ujjayi breathing for 20 breaths. Notice the sound 'So' on the inhale and the sound 'Ham' on the exhale. This simple exercise develops calm and awareness and dissolves anxiety.

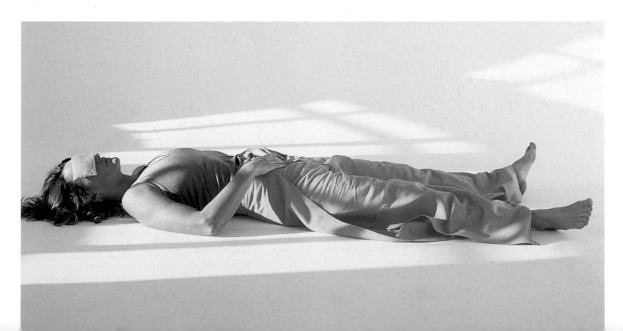

Glossary

Apana: One of the five vital energies, apana is associated with descending energy and presides over the eliminative functions of the body.

Asana: The general name for body positions in yoga.

Bandha: A psycho-muscular lock, which redirects the flow of prana (energy) in the body. There are three main bandhas – mula, uddiyana and jalandhara, but the combination of all three can make a fourth, maha.

Chakra: A vortex of energy existing at the interface between the body and mind. Chakras have associated links in the physical body through various endocrine glands, nerve plexuses, organs and the brain and spinal cord.

Chi: In Chinese medicine, chi is the life or energy force – similar to prana – that flows freely along meridians in the body in a healthy person, but which is weakened or blocked in poor health.

Dosha: In Ayurveda there are three doshas: vata, pitta, and kapha. Each person's constitution can be described in terms of one or a combination of these three and the correct balancing of doshas leads to good health.

Guna: In the Ayurvedic system, there are three qualities of nature, called gunas, that influence the mental state: rajas (energy), tamas (inertia) and sattwa (clarity or light).

Hatha yoga: Meaning the union of the sun (*Ha*) and moon (*tha*), Hatha is a branch of yoga designed to regulate energy in the body and mind.

Ida: Ida refers to the left nerve channel (nadi) through the body. It corresponds to the moon and calm, passive energy.

Kapalbhati: An air-cleansing purification process (shatkarma) that clears the frontal region of the brain, bringing clarity and illumination.

Kosha: Each person is said to have five koshas ('sheaths'). These interacting and overlapping layers of energy form the complete spiritual, mental and physical nature of the personality. Each kosha signifies a more refined dimension of consciousness.

Kriyas: Any number of techniques that energize, cleanse or purify the body.

Kundalini: In Tantra, this is the dormant potential and spiritual life force located at the base of the spine. In Sanskrit it means serpent power.

Makko-Ho: Six stretches, similar to yoga poses, but designed to stimulate and rebalance chi along the meridians and associated with the five elements (water, wood, fire, earth and metal) in traditional Chinese medicine.

Mantra: A sacred syllable or word repeated in meditation or prayer with the aim of expanding one's awareness.

Meridians: In traditional Chinese medicine, meridians are the channels in the body through which chi energy flows. There are twelve main meridians, six yin and six yang, and each relates to one of organs.

Mudra: Literally meaning 'gesture', mudras are physical, mental and psychic attitudes that express and channel pranic energy and which can open the doors of perception.

Nadis: Nadis, meaning 'conduits' or 'arteries', are channels through which prana flows. The three main nadis are ida, pingala and sushumna.

Nauli: A muscular contraction and shatkarma of the abdomen, which regenerates and stimulates the gastrointestinal system.

Neti: Jala neti is a shatkarma technique of cleansing the nasal passages by alternating the flow of water in the nostrils, preferably using a neti pot.

Pingala: Pingala refers to the right nerve channel (nadi). It corresponds to the sun and active energy.

Prana: The vital life force, similar to chi. It is also one of the five vital energies, responsible for absorption and related to ascending energy.

Pranayama: Breathing techniques that regulate and balance energy.

Samadhi: The state of supreme union, where concentration becomes one with the object of concentration.

Samana: The name of one of the five main pranas, responsible for bringing nourishment and balance to the body.

Samskara: A Sanskrit word indicating the impression left by a thought or action; a latent tendency or habit.

Shambhavi mudra: A yoga gesture which focuses at the space on the brow between the eyes.

Shatkarma: Six hatha purification practices that remove toxins and impurities from the body. They are normally performed under the guidance of a guru or teacher.

Siddhasana: A meditative seating posture in which the left heel presses the perineum. It is also known as the 'perfect pose'.

Sukhasana: A comfortable cross-legged pose, also called 'easy pose'.

Sushumna nadi: The pranic channel between ida and pingala, which rises from the bottom of the spinal cord.

Udana: The name of one of the five main pranas and the one connected with the expulsion of air and sound.

Ujjayi: A deep breathing technique that produces a light sonorous sound. It creates an awareness of a polarity in the breath – inhalation is accompanied by upward energy, while the exhalation has a descending energy.

Vayus: The five functions or patterns of prana – prana, apana, samana, udana and vyana.

Vinyasa: The order in which postures are sequenced, so as to have different effects on the internal functioning of the body as well as spiritual benefits.

Vyana: One of the five vital energies, connecting and coordinating all powers and involved with the senses.

Yantra: An aid in meditation, taking the form of either a symbolic pictorial diagram or a numerological one.

Yoga nidra: Translated as 'yogic sleep' this is a state between sleep and wakefulness, where contact with the subconscious and unconscious occurs.

Index Main references are indicated in bold.

Bibliography

Bays, Brandon, *The Journey*, Harper Collins, 1999.

Buddhananda, Chela, with Swami Satyananada Saraswati, *Moola Bandha: The Master Key*, Bihar School of Yoga, 1978.

Capra, Fritjof, *The Turning Point*, Flamingo, 1983.

Capra, Frijof, *The Web of Life: A New Synthesis of Mind and Matter*, Flamingo, 1997.

Cochrane, Jennifer, *An Illustrated History of Medicine*, Tiger, 1996.

Coulter, David, *Anatomy of Hatha Yoga: A Manual for Students, Teachers and Practitioners*, Himalayan Institute, 2002.

Dubos, Rene, *Man Adapting*, Yale University Press, 1980.

Erasmus, Udo, *Fats That Heal, Fats That Kill*, Alive Books, 1995.

Hirschi, Gertrud. *Mudras: Yogas in Your Hands*, Weiser Books, 2000.

Kraftsow, Gary, *Yoga For Wellness*, Arkana, 1999.

Kraftsow, Gary, *Yoga for Transformation*, Arkana, 2002.

Larsen, William, *Human Embryology*, Churchill Livingstone, 1997.

Margota, Roberto, *The Story of Medicine*, Golden Press, 1968.

Mehta, Mira, *Health Through Yoga: Simple Practice Routines and A Guide to the Ancient Teachings*, Harper Collins, 2002.

Moyers, Bill, *Healing and the Mind*, Doubleday, 1993.

Netter, Frank H., *Atlas of Human Anatomy*, Icon Learning Systems, 2003.

Netter, Frank H., *The CIBA Collection of Medical Illustrations: Endocrine System and Selected Metabolic Diseases*, CIBA, 1979.

Peters, David and Anne Woodham, *Complete Guide to Integrative Medicine: Combining the Best of Natural and Conventional Care*, Dorling Kindersley, 2000.

Radinsky, Leonard, *The Evolution of Vertebrate Design*, University of Chicago Press, 1987.

Rama, Swami, and Rudolph Ballentine, MD, *Yoga and Psychotherapy: The Evolution of Consciousness*, Himalayan Institute, 1998.

Rolf, Ida P., *Rolfing: Reestablishing Structural Alignment and Integration of the Human Body for Vitality and Wellbeing*, Inner Traditions, 1992.

Saraswati, Swami Satyananda, *Yoga Nidra*, Nesma Books, 2003.

Saraswati, Swami Satyananda, *Yoga and Cardiovascular Management*, Yoga Publications Trust, 2001.

Saunders, J.B. and Charles O'Malley, eds., *The Illustrations from the Works of Andreas Vesalius of Brussels*, Dover Publications, 1973.

Shankardevananda, Swami, *The Practices of Yoga for the Digestive System*, Yoga Publications Trust, 2003.

Shankardevananda, Swami, *Yoga on Hypertension*, Nesma Books, 1998.

Shankardevananda, Swami, *Yoga Management of Asthma and Diabetes*, Yoga Publications Trust, 2002.

Suplee, Curt, *Milestones of Science*, National Geographic Books, 2000.

Tortora, G.J. and N.P. Anagnostakos, *Principles of Anatomy and Physiology*, John Wiley, 2002.

Trattler, Ross, *Better Health Through Natural Healing: How to Get Well Without Drugs or Surgery*, Hinkler Books, 2004.

Wicks, K., *Key Moments in Science and Technology: From the Wheel to the Web*, Hamlyn, 1999.

Acknowledgements

Acknowledgements from Liz Lark
I would like to thank Sujata Banerjee, Lee Brindell and Tara Lee for their time and energies modelling on the photo shoot. A big thank you goes to Clare Park for her superb photographs and thanks, too, to Lisa Dyer, the editor and initiator of the project. I would also like to thank all the teachers I have had through the years, for diverse approaches to yoga in order to fit individual needs. And finally I would like to thank my co-author, Tim Goullet, for his expertise and profound knowledge.

Acknowledgements from Tim Goullet
The best teachers always leave a lasting impression on you. In my case, these two teachers continue to do so. Firstly, I would like to thank my osteopathic teacher (who is so much more than just that) for sharing his unique approach to bodywork, along with an illuminating academic cocktail of embryology and physiology to name but a few. Secondly, I would like to thank my karate instructor, Hanshi Bernard Creton, for nurturing my interest in physical movement through his many years of inspirational teaching, always managing to bring theory alive in the practical domain. I would also like to thank my parents for their support and encouragement during my years both in and out of education. Finally, I would like to thank Liz Lark for giving me the opportunity to co-author my first book and to share knowledge from our respective fields.